Core Laboratory Technologies in Clinical Immunology

Core Laboratory Technologies in Clinical Immunology

EDITED BY

ROBERT R. RICH
Dean and Professor Emeritus
School of Medicine
University of Alabama at Birmingham
Birmingham, Alabama

ELSEVIER

ELSEVIER

3251 Riverport Lane
St. Louis, Missouri 63043

Core Laboratory Technologies in Clinical Immunology ISBN: 978-0-323-66149-2

Publisher: Dolores Meloni
Acquisition Editor: Robin R. Carter
Editorial Project Manager: Tracy Tufaga
Production Project Manager: Poulouse Joseph
Cover Designer: Miles Hitchen

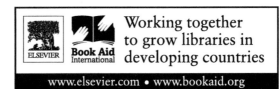

List of Contributors

Roshini Sarah Abraham, PhD
Consultant, Professor of Medicine and Laboratory
    Medicine and Pathology
Laboratory Medicine and Pathology
Mayo Clinic
Rochester, MN, United States

John W. Belmont, MD, PhD
Professor (Adjunct)
Molecular and Human Genetics, and Pediatrics
Baylor College of Medicine
Houston, TX, United States

Javier Chinen, MD, PhD
Associate Professor
Pediatrics, Allergy, Immunology, Rheumatology
    Section
Baylor College of Medicine
Houston, TX, United States

Clinic Chief
The David Clinic, Allergy and Immunology
Texas Children's Hospital — The Woodlands
The Woodlands, TX, United States

Thomas A. Fleisher, MD
Executive Vice President
American Academy of Allergy
    Asthma and Immunology
Milwaukee, WI;
Scientist Emeritus,
NIH Clinical Center
National Institutes of Health
Bethesda, MD, United States

Robert G. Hamilton, PhD, DABMLI
Professor
Medicine and Pathology
Johns Hopkins University School of Medicine
Baltimore, MD, United States

Douglas B. Kuhns, PhD
Principal Scientist
Neutrophil Monitoring Lab, Applied/Developmental
    Research Directorate
Leidos Biomedical Research, Inc.
Frederick, MD, United States

Robert L. Nussbaum, MD
Chief Medical Officer
Invitae Inc.
San Francisco, CA, United States

Former Holly Smith Professor
Medicine
University of California San Francisco
San Francisco, CA, United States

Joao B. Oliveira, MD, PhD
Research Director
Instituto de Medicina Integral Prof.
    Fernando Figueira - IMIP
Recife, PE, Brazil

Debra Long Priel, MS
Clinical Services Program
Leidos Biomedical Research, Inc.
Frederick, MD, United States

Mary E. Paul, MD
Associated Professor
Immunology, Allergy and Rheumatology Division
Department of Pediatrics
Baylor College of Medicine
Houston, TX, United States

Jennifer M. Puck, MD
Professor
Pediatrics
University of California San Francisco
San Francisco, CA, United States

Robert R. Rich, MD
Dean and Professor Emeritus
Medicine
School of Medicine
University of Alabama at Birmingham
Birmingham, Alabama

Sergio D. Rosenzweig, MD, PhD
Chief, Immunology Service
Department of Laboratory Medicine
NIH Clinical Center
National Institutes of Health
Bethesda, MD, United States

William T. Shearer, MD, PhD
Professor of Pediatrics and Pathology and
    Immunology, Distinguished Service Professor
Immunology Allergy Rheumatology
Baylor College of Medicine
Houston, TX, United States

Chief
Allergy and Immunology Service
Texas Children's Hospital
Houston, TX, United States

Preface

The fifth edition of the comprehensive textbook *Clinical Immunology: Principles and Practice* was very recently published. Since the first edition, its target audience has been predominantly clinicians who directly care for patients with immunological diseases. There are, however, substantial numbers of physicians and scientists who are not involved in direct patient care, but whose professional expertise is profoundly important to the overall management of patients with the diseases that define clinical immunology. This population of scientists and physicians includes clinical pathologists and PhD immunologists who are involved in translational research utilizing the essential laboratory tools of the clinical immunologist.

This reasoning that led to a conclusion that a much smaller book, specifically focused on *Core Technologies in Clinical Immunology,* could fill an important niche. To that end, Elsevier content strategist Robin Carter and I examined the comprehensive textbook for chapters that might concisely provide such information, without the unnecessary content relevant to physicians primarily involved in direct patient care.

The chapters so identified included two on the approaches and techniques of genomic evaluation, the critical technology of flow cytometry, the *in vitro* assessment of lymphocyte and neutrophil function, tools for *in vitro* study of human allergic diseases and the laboratory evaluation of patients with suspected immunodeficiency. Additionally two appendices from the comprehensive textbook have been included: 1) the expression and characteristics of many CD molecules that define subsets of cells of the immune system; 2) clinical laboratory reference values of primary interest to clinical immunologists. These chapters are largely replicates of relevant chapters in the comprehensive book, although some content relevant only to physicians involved directly in patient care has been deleted. Other edits provide additional references and updates of information published since the preparation of that book. I hope that you find it useful.

Robert R. Rich, MD

Contents

CHAPTER 1

Genomics in Human Immunology

ROBERT L. NUSSBAUM • JENNIFER M. PUCK

The completion of the Human Genome Project in 2003, 50 years after the landmark 1953 publication of the double-helical structure of DNA by James Watson and Francis Crick, is correctly deemed a major milestone in modern biology. The sequence provided a first comprehensive and accurate view of the genetic makeup of humans, with a low error rate and only a few hundred gaps of indeterminate sequence. The first detailed picture of the structure of a composite human genome is for human genetics what Vesalius's publication of a consensus structure of the human body, *De humani corporis fabrica*, was for anatomy. And, like Vesalius's work, it continues to serve as a foundation for further scientific discovery in areas such as genetic variation, gene function, human physiology, and the genetic basis for disease. The years following the completion of the first human genome sequencing have seen progress in all of these areas.

Key Concepts

The sequence of the human genome and catalogue of extensive genome variation among humans have revolutionized our approach to heritable immune disorders.

Genomic variation between humans and other species illuminates conserved areas that are critical for normal function of gene products.

A variety of types of DNA variations are recognized, including single nucleotide changes, insertions, or deletions of a few to many nucleotides, copy number variants, and structural variants.

Interpretation of the significance of an observed variant in DNA sequence may require consideration of its location, frequency in the population, inheritance in a family, and specific effect on the resulting gene product.

GENOME ANNOTATION

A consensus sequence of the human genome is only the first step in furthering our understanding of normal biological functions and how mutations lead to abnormal functions that cause disease. The

Human Genome Project has now matured into a number of important basic and applied research areas: *(i)* acquiring a comprehensive catalogue of human variation and the impact of such variation on phenotype, including disorders of human development; *(ii)* comparing the genomes of humans with those of other organisms, including model organisms and human ancestors; and *(iii)* learning how to interpret all the sequence elements within the genome, not just the codons. Even now, over a dozen years after "completion" of the human genome sequence, a complete, accurate, and single contiguous stretch representing a reference human haploid genome is still being constructed, and updated versions of the genome sequence continue to be released. As described below, the greatest challenges to completing the human genome sequence are posed by regions that contain segmental duplications of nearly the same sequence.[1]

HUMAN VARIATION

The first publicly available human genome sequence was constructed from a small number of individuals. Nonetheless, the "reference" human genome sequence available at public websites is a consensus, composite haploid sequence and not the sequence of any one individual. It is neither a "normal" genome nor a "control" genome; instead, it serves as a reference, providing a universally available sequence against which the genomes of other individuals, as well as other species, can be compared and any differences ("variants") determined. Even before the original human genome sequence was completed, the need to discover as broad a range of human variations as possible in populations from around the world was clearly recognized to be essential if we were to begin to understand how variations in the genome lead to differences in phenotypic variations in traits and disease susceptibilities. The first concerted efforts to catalogue human genetic diversity after completion of the Human Genome Project was the dbSNP (database of single

Core Laboratory Technologies in Clinical Immunology. https://doi.org/10.1016/B978-0-323-66149-2.00001-3

nucleotide polymorphisms) project, followed by the 1000 Genomes project. These initial catalogues that surveyed the extent of variation in both the coding and the noncoding portions of the genome have been supplemented enormously by more comprehensive sequencing efforts, which produced the NHLBI GO Exome Sequencing Project (ESP) and Exome Aggregation Consortium (ExAC). These projects focus on variation within exomes of hundreds of thousands of individuals and have made a vast number of variants and their frequency publicly available to researchers and clinicians worldwide.

Variants can be classified as rare or common (polymorphic) according to their *frequency* in a population under study. Any variant present in >2% of the population (*i.e.,* constituting >1% of the alleles at any locus in that population) is arbitrarily designated as polymorphic. With the advent of comprehensive DNA sequencing of larger and larger numbers of people from across the globe, it has become clear that most variants (85%) at any one base pair (bp) or segment of the genome have allele frequencies substantially below the 1% cutoff for being a polymorphism and are, instead, considered rare, sometimes restricted to a single ethnic group or even a single kindred.[2]

DNA variation can also be classified according to the *type* of DNA change seen in the variant (Table 1.1).

Single nucleotide variants (SNVs), insertion/deletion (indel) variants, copy number variants (CNVs), and structural variants (SVs) can have different consequences, depending on their location and the number and identity of nucleotides affected.

The simplest and most common of all variants are SNVs, in which one nucleotide in the reference sequence is substituted by another. A locus characterized by an SNV usually has only two alleles, corresponding to the more common (major allele) and less common (minor allele) bases found at that particular location in the genome, although, theoretically, four alleles at any one base position are possible. SNVs are observed on average once every 1000 bp in the genome but are not distributed evenly throughout and are most often not equally frequent throughout all populations. Most SNVs are found in the 98% of genomic sequence that is not within exons, including the ∼20% of the genome inside genes, in introns, with the remaining ∼80% between genes. Nonetheless, many SNVs are in coding portions of genes and other known functional elements in the genome. Just under half of these do not alter the predicted amino acid sequence of the encoded protein and are thus termed *synonymous,* whereas the remainder do alter the amino acid sequence and are said to be *nonsynonymous.* Other SNVs introduce or change a

TABLE 1.1
DNA Variants

Type	Description	Ability to Detect	Frequency in an Individual
Single nucleotide variants (SNVs)	A sequence change where, compared with a reference sequence, one nucleotide is substituted for another nucleotide	High	3 000 000–4 000 000
Deletion or duplication (Del/Dup) variants	A sequence change involving between 2 and ∼1000 base pairs (bp) in which reference nucleotides are either not present (deleted) or are duplicated and inserted directly 3' of the original copy of the sequence	Moderate	1 000 000?
Insertion/deletion (Indel) variants	A sequence change involving between 2 and ∼1000 bp in which one or more reference nucleotides are replaced by one or more other nucleotides and is not an SNV or SV	Moderate	
Copy number variants (CNVs)	Del/Dup or Indel arbitrarily set as larger than ∼1000 bp	Difficult	
Structural variants (SVs)		Very difficult	

From Human Variome Society, Sequence Variant Nomenclature. 2016. Available at: http://varnomen.hgvs.org.

stop codon, and yet others alter a known splice site; such SNVs are expected to have significant functional consequences.

A second general class of variation is the result of insertion and/or deletion of reference sequence ranging from 1 up to an arbitrary cutoff of ~300—1000 bp, that is, a variant size that can be detected by the most commonly used next-generation sequencing (NGS) technology. When reference nucleotides are simply deleted or duplicated, the variant is referred to as a "del/dup." When reference sequence has some nucleotides deleted and *replaced* by other inserted sequence, the variant is referred to as an "indel." Approximately half of all del/dups are referred to as "simple" because they have only two alleles—that is, the presence or absence of the inserted or deleted segment. Each individual is known to carry hundreds of thousands of indels, but this estimate is suspected to be too low, and a corrected estimate for indels per individual may be upward of a million.[3] Up to 30—40% of actual indels are likely to be missing from catalogues because of the technical difficulties of distinguishing many indels from sequencing errors using the current sequencing technologies.[4]

Some del/dup variants are multiallelic because of variable numbers of the identical segment of DNA inserted in tandem at a particular location, thereby constituting what is referred to as a *microsatellite* (also referred to as a *short tandem repeat* [STR]). Microsatellites are segments of DNA composed of units of 2, 3, or 4 nucleotides, such as TGTG...TG, CAACAA...CAA, or AAATAAAT...AAAT. The units are repeated between two and a few dozen times at a particular site in the genome. Some variation in microsatellite length is common enough to constitute a *polymorphism*, defined as an allele or alleles other than the reference sequence, found in ≥2% of the population. Many tens of thousands of polymorphic microsatellites are known to exist throughout the human genome. There are, however, STR DNA segments present within exons or splice junctions of >90% of genes associated with human disease. They rarely, but famously, can expand to become hundreds or thousands of nucleotides long, thereby causing such human disorders as fragile X syndrome or Huntington disease. Even without expansion, STRs within exons, some of which may be as small as 9—25 bp, have an outsized impact on the frequency of human disease, since they confer a five- to sixfold increase in the frequency of rare disease-causing indel mutations compared with neighboring exon sequences that do not contain an STR.[5]

One subclass of indel variants arises from mobile elements. Nearly half of the human genome sequence consists of families of repetitive elements dispersed throughout the genome, of which the two most common are the *Alu* (a short interspersed nuclear element [SINE], usually about 300 bp) and LINE (long interspersed nuclear element) families of repeats. Although most of the copies of these repeats are stationary, some of them contribute to human genetic diversity through *retrotransposition*, a process that involves insertion of a DNA segment generated through transcription of an *Alu* or LINE element into an RNA that is then reverse-transcribed into a DNA sequence that is inserted into the genomic DNA. Each mobile element indel consists of two alleles, one with and one without the inserted mobile element. Mobile element polymorphisms are found on all human chromosomes; although most are found in nongenic regions of the genome, a small proportion exist within genes. At least 5000 of them are known to be frequent enough to be polymorphisms, and insertion frequencies of >10% occur in various populations; other mobile elements are rare and have been implicated in causing insertional mutations in human disease genes. As with other indels, difficulties with sequencing, in particular the challenges posed to NGS by repetitive DNA, result in underestimation of *Alu* and LINE indels throughout the genome.[3]

Another important type of human variation includes CNVs. These consist of variations in the number of copies of segments of the genome that are larger than those involved in indels and range in size from 1000 bp to many hundreds of kilobase (kb) pairs. Variants larger than 500 kb are found in 5—10% of individuals in the general population, whereas variants encompassing more than a million bases (1 Mb) are found in 1—2%.[6] Smaller CNVs, in particular, may have only two alleles (*i.e.*, the presence or absence of a segment), similar to indels. Larger CNVs tend to have multiple alleles because of the presence of different numbers of copies of a segment of DNA in tandem. The content of any two human genomes can differ by as much as 50—100 Mb as a result of copy number differences at CNV loci, compared with some 3—4 Mb of differences because of SNVs and indels. Thus simply on the basis of the number of nucleotides involved in the variation, CNVs represent vastly more human variation than do SNVs or indels.

Not only are CNVs a very significant contributor to human variation and disease,[7] the areas of the genome where they are found are often the sites of segmental duplications,[8] some of the most difficult regions in which to develop an accurate reference sequence. Segmental duplications are ubiquitous throughout the genome. It is difficult to construct an accurate contiguous genome sequence in regions of segmental duplications because the most widely used massively parallel sequencing technologies generate only short reads of a few hundred base pairs and therefore may not be able to differentiate between the sequences of nearly identical DNA segments using unique DNA that flanks them. The assembly algorithms, which always try to create the simplest assembly possible, may consider two nearly identical segments of DNA that have been duplicated in the genome, but differ at a few locations in their sequence, to be the same sequence and collapse them into a single segment of DNA. The fixed sequence differences between the duplicated segments are incorrectly interpreted as polymorphic differences between two alleles of a nonduplicated locus instead of being real sequence differences between different copies of duplicated DNA. The fact that there is a segmental duplication is therefore overlooked. Conversely, the sequence of a unique DNA segment with many SNVs compared with the reference may be incorrectly interpreted as having come from distinct but highly similar duplicated segments, leading to the supposition that there are paralogues or duplicated segments. As a result, segmental duplications are liable to both false-negative and false-positive representations in the human genome assembly. CNVs are particularly difficult to detect and interpret if the number of segments in the reference is incorrect or ambiguous.

Many CNVs include genes, from one up to several dozens; thus CNVs are frequently implicated in diseases that result from altered gene dosage.[7] One well-known human immunological multisystem disorder, DiGeorge syndrome, is caused by a deletion CNV that occurs *de novo* in about 1 in 5000 individuals. When a CNV is more frequent, it represents a background of common polymorphism that must be understood if to properly interpret alterations in copy number observed in patients. As with all DNA variations, the significance of different CNV alleles in health and in disease susceptibility is the subject of intensive investigation.

The most common SVs in the human genome sequence are inversions, which differ in size from a few base pairs to large regions of the genome (up to several million bases) that can be present in either of two orientations in the genomes of different individuals.[8] As with CNVs, inversions are usually flanked by regions of sequence homology, which indicates that recombination of these homologous regions is likely involved in the origin of the inversions.[7,8] Most inversions do not involve gain or loss of DNA; in this case, the two alleles corresponding to the two orientations can achieve substantial frequencies in the general population. Such inversions can, however, cause significant gains or losses of DNA in the offspring of inversion carriers because of aberrant recombination during meiosis, leading to serious syndromes brought about by chromosomal imbalance. Furthermore, if inversions interfere with normal gene expression by disrupting a gene or altering the physical relationship between a gene and its regulatory elements, it may be detrimental to health.[9,10]

CLINICAL IMPACT OF HUMAN VARIATION

One of the greatest challenges facing human geneticists is linking variation to phenotype.[11] The significance for the health of the vast majority of variants of any type is unknown, and yet this knowledge is essential if we are to apply genomics to clinical care. The impact of variants ranges from completely benign to highly pathogenic, the latter causing devastating disorders of the immune system that may occur as new mutation dominants or as autosomal recessively inherited syndromes. Even common polymorphic variants may affect health or longevity, although their being common means that they are likely to produce a relatively subtle alteration of disease susceptibility rather than directly cause a serious illness.[12] Working out the functional impact of human variation will occupy genomics researchers for many years to come. An essential component of this work is to make databases of genetic variants and their impact on human health available to the research and clinical communities, as is being done with the ClinVar database hosted by the National Library of Medicine in the United States and the Leiden Open-source Variation Database (LOVD).[13-15]

COMPARATIVE GENOMICS

Evolution at work is nowhere better illustrated than in the field of comparative genomics, which deals with similarities in the sequence, structure, and chromosomal location of genes between different species whose evolutionary paths diverged from a few years ago to many hundreds of millions of years ago. Direct sequence comparison has revealed that an enormous number of human proteins have orthologues (genes derived from a common ancestor) in other organisms, ranging from 87% in chimps to 79% in

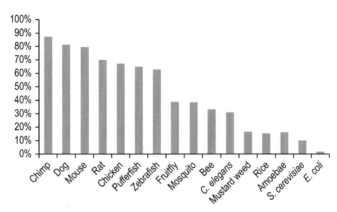

FIG. 1.1 Homology Between Genes of Humans and Those of Multiple Other Organisms. Comparisons were made by calculating gene homology or similarity between reference protein sequences from human and another species, with homology considered present when the probability of an interspecies match by chance alone was <10^{-30}. (Reproduced with permission from Nussbaum R. Human genomics and development. In: Epstein CJ, Erickson RP, Wynshaw-Boris A, editors. Inborn errors of development. New York: Oxford University Press; 2008.)

mice, 63% in zebrafish, 39% in the fruit fly (*Drosophila melanogaster*), and 31% in the nematode (*Caenorhabditis elegans*) (Fig. 1.1). The study of the human genome and the genomic basis for human disease has benefited from studies done in other organisms, particularly mice, in which many decades of inbreeding and gene manipulation have permitted study of the genes and underlying mechanisms by which mutations responsible for immune defects lead to phenotypes. Mouse models of immunity have been highly relevant and informative for humans.

However, orthologous genes may serve different functions in different species; therefore one cannot assume that a disease-causing mutation in humans will cause a similar defect when its orthologue is similarly mutated in mice, and vice versa. For example, the V(D)J recombination activating genes *RAG1* and *RAG2* in humans and *Rag1* and *Rag2* in mice appear to have identical functions, with knockout mice showing the same inability to recombine T- and B-lymphocyte antigen receptor genes as humans with RAG1 or RAG2 deficient severe combined immunodeficiency (SCID).[16] As a result, the lymphocyte profile in both species is absent in T and B cells with normal natural killer (NK) cells, referred to as T$^-$B$^-$NK$^+$ SCID. A contrasting situation occurs in other SCID genotypes. For example, humans lacking the common γ chain (γc) of receptors for interleukin-2 (IL-2) and other cytokines, caused by mutations in the X-linked gene *IL2RG*, have SCID in which T and NK cells are absent but nonfunctional B cells are present in normal to high numbers, T$^-$B$^+$NK$^-$ SCID. Mice

with the orthologous gene *Il2rg* mutated or removed can make T cells but have no B cells, which gives them a T$^+$B$^-$NK$^-$ phenotype.[17]

Genes other than *IL2RG* alone must be responsible for this difference between species. Such genes, known as *modifiers*, have not yet been identified. Notably, different strains of mice can also have important phenotypic differences in the presence of a single gene mutation under study; some strains, for example, nonobese diabetic (NOD) and Murphy Roths Large (MRL) mice are highly prone to developing autoimmunity, while others such as C57BL/6 (B6) are resistant.[18]

FUNCTIONAL GENOMICS

Immediately after the Human Genome Project was declared to have been completed in 2003, an important follow-on project was launched to identify the functional segments of DNA, particularly portions in the 98−99% lying outside of the coding exons of genes, for which there was no simple sequence code that could be understood the way the triplet codon code can be read. This project, termed ENCODE (for "encyclopedia of DNA elements"), began as a pilot project to identify functional elements in 1% of the genome, but it was quickly expanded to include the entire human genome as well as the genomes of model organisms.[19] Before ENCODE, estimates were that 3−8% of the human genome had some role in function, given that this fraction of the genome appeared to be highly conserved among species with only very limited variation. This

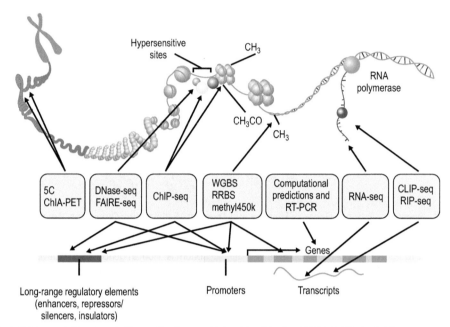

FIG. 1.2 Transcriptional and Chromatin Assays Being Used in the ENCODE Project. The assays can be used to identify regions of the genome involved in the regulation of gene expression. (With permission from https://www.encodeproject.org.)

estimate was clearly too low, as it did not take into account rapidly evolving functional elements or those restricted to particular evolutionary lineages. This estimate also did not include segments of DNA that were too small to show conservation with statistical significance, nor did it include the functional elements in repetitive DNA that are not reliably scored as being evolutionarily conserved.

Since the same genome is present but functions differently in different cells of an individual, ENCODE used a number of different tissues for its studies (Fig. 1.2). A comprehensive catalogue of every segment of DNA that is transcribed into RNA in any tissue, including all splice isoforms, was required, including RNAs that code for a protein or are noncoding and function in gene regulation. ENCODE is analyzing not only total whole-cell RNAs but also those located in the nucleus or cytosol because subcellular localization of RNAs is important in how RNA is processed and functions. Other assays for functionality of segments of DNA include biochemical evidence, such as identifying *(i)* segments of DNA located in chromatin loops that allow chromatin—chromatin interaction; *(ii)* regions of open chromatin, which are accessible to transcription; *(iii)* motifs that bind transcription factors; *(iv)* regions that are associated with histones that have been modified to either promote or suppress transcription; and *(v)* regions with differential methylation of cytosine residues in different tissues, with methylation being associated with inactivity.

Now, approximately 15 years into the project, ENCODE has created a large database of more than 4 million functional regions of the genome. Mostly on the basis of biochemical evidence, it has been estimated that 80% of the genome *may* be of functional significance,[20] but this estimate is probably too high and has been strongly criticized. For example, evidence of transcription of a segment does not necessarily mean that the transcript plays any functional role, nor is it likely to be true that the millions of vestigial repetitive DNA sequences that are undergoing mutation without any apparent selection could have important functional roles.[21] A more stringent threshold for ascribing a functional role to DNA segments (*i.e.*, direct effect on gene expression and phenotype of at least one human cell type) reduces that fraction to the range of 10—20%. Much more research will be needed before the ENCODE project delivers its final assessment of the fraction of the human genome that plays a role in gene regulation—that is, in how different cells use their genomes.[22]

APPLYING HUMAN GENOMICS TO UNDERSTANDING DISORDERS OF THE HUMAN IMMUNE SYSTEM

Genome research has provided geneticists with a catalogue of all known human genes, knowledge of their location and structure, and an ever-growing list of variants in DNA sequences found among individuals in different populations. In the past, geneticists followed two approaches to identifying the genetic basis for human disorders. The first approach, linkage analysis, is *family based* (Fig. 1.3). Linkage analysis takes advantage of family pedigrees to follow the inheritance of a disease among family members and test a few hundred DNA variants distributed throughout the genome for consistent, repeated coinheritance, or segregation, with the disease. A demonstration of significant coinheritance with a *variant* or *variants* located in a particular region of the genome indicates that the disease-causing mutation is also located in a gene within or near this region. The variants showing coinheritance with the disease are usually not the variants responsible for the disorder. Marker variants need, however, to be located close enough that recombination between the marker and the gene mutation responsible for the disease is sufficiently rare that cosegregation is observed over a few generations.

The second approach, genome-wide association study (GWAS), is *population based*. A sample of affected individuals, or "cases," taken from the population, is chosen along with a matched set of unaffected "control"

individuals from the same population. Then, a large number, in the order of a million or more, variants are examined individually for an increased or decreased frequency of cases compared with controls. The alleles used to *test* for association need not be the actual variants functionally *responsible* for the disease association—in fact, it is highly unlikely this would be the case. Instead, GWAS, like linkage, depends on the vast number of marker alleles that can be tested for association to be located close enough to the alleles functionally responsible for association to have been carried along, on the same chromosome in a haplotype block, through many generations (Fig. 1.4). Association analysis does not require pedigrees and is particularly useful for complex diseases that do not show strict mendelian inheritance.[23]

Linkage analysis and association studies have limitations in investigating the genetic basis for human immunological disorders. Linkage analysis is problematic if the disorder is a rare autosomal recessive condition such that there are not enough families with two carrier parents to enable such a study; nonetheless, the increased frequency of consanguineous matings in some populations has been utilized to overcome this limitation.[24,25] Another challenge with linkage analysis is if the disorder is genetically lethal so that it is never inherited and always occurs sporadically as a result of a new mutation. Detecting an association in a case-control study is also a problem when the frequency of any particular allele associated with the disease is too

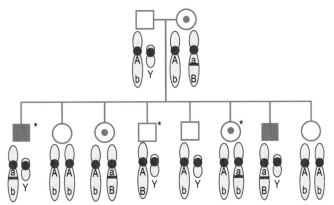

FIG. 1.3 An Example of Family-Based Linkage Analysis to Identify a Disease Gene. The pedigree of a family with X-linked severe combined immunodeficiency (SCID) caused by an *IL2RG* mutation in the proximal long arm of the X chromosome *(marked with black bar)* is shown. Affected males have filled in square; female carriers are designated by dot in the center of their symbols. Two loci, one with alleles A and a, and the other with alleles B and b, are shown in the proximal and distal long arm of the X (Xq). There are no recombinations during female meiosis between allele a and the *IL2RG* mutation in any of the eight children, while three children *(marked with asterisk)* show a recombination with the locus on the distal Xq. The father's X chromosome is passed on without any recombinations to each of his daughters and is shown on the left of each pair of X chromosomes in the daughters.

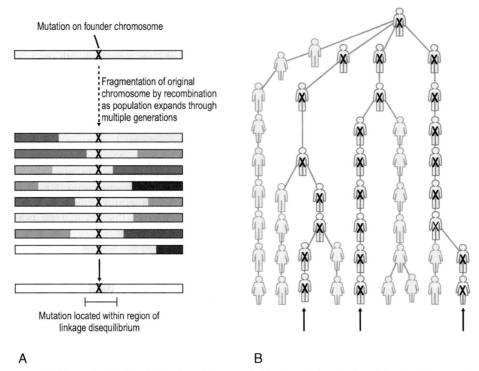

FIG. 1.4 An Example of a Population-Based Genome-Wide Association Study to Identify a Disease Gene. (A) A mutation (X) that predisposes to a disease first occurs on a chromosome with a certain set of alleles at polymorphic loci along that chromosome *(symbolized by the blue color)*. With each generation, meiotic recombination exchanges the alleles that were initially present at polymorphic loci on the "blue chromosome" for other alleles present on homologous chromosomes *(symbolized by other colors)*. Over many generations, the only alleles that remain associated with the mutation are those at loci so close to the mutant locus that recombination between them is very rare. These alleles constitute a disease-associated haplotype. (B) Affected individuals in the current generation *(arrows)* that carry the mutation **(X)** are enriched for the disease-associated haplotype *(individuals in blue)* compared with unaffected individuals. Depending on the age of the mutation and other population genetic factors, a disease-associated haplotype ordinarily spans a region of DNA of a few kilobases to a few hundred kilobases. (From Nussbaum R, McInnes RR, Willard HF. Thompson and Thompson Genetics in medicine. 8th ed. Toronto, Canada: Elsevier Canada; 2016: 177, Fig. 10.8, with permission.)

low among the cases to give a detectable association. For example, if the disorder arises from different, independent mutations and if these mutations are found on many different haplotypes in affected individuals, it may be very difficult to establish a significant association with any one variant.

When linkage and association studies are not possible, as in very rare mendelian disorders, a third approach is now available—genome sequencing. Vastly improved methods of DNA sequencing have cut the cost of sequencing six orders of magnitude over what was spent generating the Human Genome Project's reference sequence, opening up new possibilities to discover the genes and mutations responsible for rare mendelian disorders. One can generate a whole-genome sequence (WGS) or, in what has often

proven a cost-effective compromise, a sequence of only about 2% of the genome, the part containing the exons of genes, referred to as a whole-exome sequence (WES).

As an example of what is now possible, suppose that there is a family "trio" consisting of a child affected with a rare immunodeficiency and his or her parents. WES is carried out on the child and the parents, yielding typically 30-40,000 SNV, indel, and CNV differences in the child compared with the human genome reference sequence. Which of these variants would be responsible for the disease? The extraction of useful information from such a massive amount of data relies on creating a variant filtering scheme based on a variety of reasonable assumptions about likely responsible explanations for the disease.

One example of a filtering scheme that can be used to sort through these variants is shown in Fig. 1.5, in which exome sequence was performed for two parents and their offspring, two affected and one unaffected.

1. *Location with respect to protein-coding genes.* Keep variants that are within or near exons of protein-coding genes and discard variants deep within introns or intergenic regions. It is possible, of course, that the responsible mutation might lie in a noncoding RNA gene (*e.g.*, *RMRP*, the gene mutated in the immunodeficiency and dwarfing syndrome cartilage hair hypoplasia). However, these are currently more difficult to assess, and thus, as a simplifying assumption, it is reasonable to focus initially on protein-coding genes.

2. *Population frequency.* Keep rare variants from Step 1 and discard common variants with allele frequencies >0.05 (or some other arbitrary number between 0.01 and 0.1) because common variants are highly unlikely to be responsible for a disease whose population prevalence is much less than the q^2 predicted by the Hardy-Weinberg equilibrium.

3. *Deleterious nature of the mutation.* Keep variants from Step 2 that cause nonsense or nonsynonymous changes in codons within exons, cause frame-shift mutations, or alter highly conserved splice sites. Discard synonymous changes that have no predicted effect on protein function (unless there is reason to suspect that they influence splicing or expression, such as the last nucleotide of an exon, which is typically "G").

4. *Consistency with likely inheritance pattern.* If the disorder is considered most likely to be autosomal recessive, keep any variants from Step 3 for which an affected child has two variants in the same gene and each parent has one of the variants. The child need not be homozygous for the same deleterious variant but could be a compound heterozygote for two different deleterious mutations in the same gene.

In the example in Fig. 1.5, the two affected children were compound heterozygous for variants, with each parent and the unaffected sister carrying one of the variants. If there were consanguinity in the parents, the candidate genes and variants might be further filtered by requiring that the child be a true homozygote for the same mutation derived from a single common ancestor. If the autosomal recessive mode of inheritance is correct, then the parents should both be heterozygous for the variants. The disease-causing variant in a male could also be X-linked, in which case any variant found in an X-linked gene for which the mother is a heterozygote would be a candidate.

For either the autosomal or X-linked case, the disorder could be the result of a new dominant

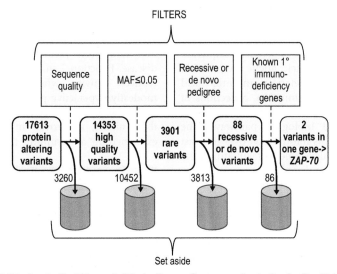

FIG. 1.5 Variant Filtering to Sort Through Whole-Exome Sequence Analysis of a Familial Disease. Protein-altering variants detected in the affected children, their unaffected sibling, and parents were first filtered by sequencing quality and allele frequency to yield a set of 88 rare, damaging, or nonsynonymous variants that fit an autosomal recessive inheritance pattern and were then candidates for causing the autoimmune disorder. This group was then further analyzed for genes involved in immune function, which brought two variants in *ZAP-70*, for which the affected children were both compound heterozygotes, to the top of the list as possible causative mutations. (Adapted from Chan et al. A novel human autoimmune syndrome caused by combined hypomorphic and activating mutations in ZAP-70. J Exp Med 2016;213:155–65, with permission.)

mutation; in this case, keep variants from Step 3 that are *de novo* changes in the child and are not present in either parent.

In the end, tens of thousands of variants can often be filtered down to a handful of SNVs, indels, or CNVs affecting a reasonable number of genes. Once the filtering reduces the number of genes and alleles to a manageable number, they can be assessed individually for other characteristics. Do any of the genes have a known function or tissue expression pattern that would be expected if it were the potential disease gene? Is the gene already implicated in other disease phenotypes, or does it have a role in pathways in which mutations are known to cause similar or different phenotypes? Finally, is the same gene mutated in other patients or in an animal model with the disease? Finding mutations in one of the candidate genes as well as in other patients would confirm that this gene was the responsible gene in the trio under study. In some cases, one gene remaining on the list in Step 4 may become a leading candidate because its involvement makes biological or genetic sense or it is known to be mutated in other affected individuals. In other cases, however, the gene responsible may turn out to be entirely unanticipated on biological grounds or may not be mutated in other affected individuals because of locus heterogeneity (*i.e.*, mutations in other as yet undiscovered genes can cause a similar disease).

Such variant assessments require extensive use of public genomic databases and software tools. These include the human genome reference sequence, databases of variants with their allelic frequencies, software that assesses how deleterious an amino acid substitution might be to gene function, collections of known disease-causing mutations, and databases of functional networks and biological pathways. The enormous expansion of this information over the past few years has played a crucial role in facilitating gene discovery of rare mendelian disorders.

In a recent report of the clinical use of WES in rare disorders,[26] 2000 individuals with a variety of disorders that had escaped diagnosis despite thorough conventional clinical evaluations underwent WES. A likely causative mutation or pair of mutations was found in 504 (25.2%). Of these mutations (of which many were severe developmental defects), half were *de novo*, not present in either parent. Also of interest was that 23 (4.6%) of these 504 patients in whom a diagnosis was made through WES had two different genetic disorders, resulting in a combined phenotype, most likely obscuring the diagnosis of either of the individual disorders had they been present alone.

In some cases, the difficulty in making a diagnosis was the result of there being a mutation in a gene, previously unknown to cause human disease, but implicated by finding mutations that fit the inheritance pattern (*de novo* dominant or autosomal recessive), and then later confirmed by finding other mutations in phenotypically similar patients. In others, the gene involved had been previously described, but not in association with the phenotype for which the patient was undergoing diagnostic exome analysis. An example is, two children affected with an undiagnosed autoimmune syndrome consisting of early-onset bullous pemphigoid, nephritis, autoimmune antifactor VIII hemophilia, and inflammatory bowel disease. WES was performed for both children, their unaffected sister, and both unaffected parents.[27] Eighty-eight genes were found in which the two affected children were compound heterozygotes for two different rare mutations, whereas the unaffected sister and both parents were carriers for only one of the two mutations found in the children. Of these, only one gene was known to have any immunological function: *ZAP70*, previously known to be mutated in combined immunodeficiency but not with strictly autoimmune disease of this type (see Fig. 1.5). Both affected children were compound heterozygotes for two missense mutations, p.R192W and p.R360P, in *ZAP70*. The mother carried the R192W allele, whereas the father and unaffected sister carried the R360P allele. Neither mutation had been reported previously, nor were they near mutations in the same gene that had been previously associated with human disease. Functional studies revealed the p.R192W had reduced activity, whereas the R360P encoded a modestly hyperactive protein because of disruption of an autoinhibitory mechanism. The combination of these alleles, as proven in laboratory studies, fully explained the autoimmune phenotype.

> ### On the Horizon
>
> As the costs of deep sequencing fall, examination of whole-genome sequence should allow for examination of noncoding regulatory regions.
>
> Data storage and computer speed will need to be improved to handle 50-fold more data from each individual.
>
> New analytical paradigms for the analysis of variation in noncoding DNA and the interpretation of DNA variants that are not clearly associated with deleterious effects will be required.
>
> Proving causality of new gene variants in primary immunodeficiencies will depend on future cataloguing of deleterious mutations in each gene and on molecular studies of the direct effects of the variants.

Since the application of WGS or WES to rare mendelian disorders was first described in 2009, hundreds of such disorders have been studied and the causative mutations found in nearly 500 previously unrecognized disease genes.[28] The pace of discovery will only increase, and we can anticipate that the number of known mendelian disorders, including those characterized by primary immunodeficiency and/or autoimmunity, will grow over coming years. It has been predicted that the genetic basis for every human single gene disorder will be elucidated in the near future. However, the genetic basis for complex disorders that show increased familial occurrence, and yet are not single gene disorders and do not follow mendelian inheritance, remains elusive and will require another leap in technology and genetic analytical tools to be fully unraveled. The data being generated through human and model organism genomics will certainly aid in the elucidation of these more challenging disorders of the human immune system. New tools available to immunologists and geneticists will open great opportunities for discovery and understanding of genetic disorders of immunity, which, in turn, will deepen our knowledge of immune system networks.

REFERENCES

1. Steinberg KM, et al. Single haplotype assembly of the human genome from a hydatidiform mole. *Genome Res.* 2014;24:2066−2076.
2. Gonzaga-Jauregui C, Lupski JR, Gibbs RA. Human genome sequencing in health and disease. *Annu Rev Med.* 2012;63: 35−61.
3. Jiang Y, Turinsky AL, Brudno M. The missing indels: an estimate of indel variation in a human genome and analysis of factors that impede detection. *Nucleic Acids Res.* 2015; 43:7217−7228.
4. Huddleston J, Eichler EE. An incomplete understanding of human genetic variation. *Genetics.* 2016;202:1251−1254.
5. Madsen BE, Villesen P, Wiuf C. Short tandem repeats in human exons: a target for disease mutations. *BMC Genomics.* 2008;9:410.
6. McCarroll SA, et al. Common deletion polymorphisms in the human genome. *Nat Genet.* 2006;38:86−92.
7. Stankiewicz P, Lupski JR. Structural variation in the human genome and its role in disease. *Annu Rev Med.* 2010;61: 437−455.
8. Carvalho CM, Lupski JR. Mechanisms underlying structural variant formation in genomic disorders. *Nat Rev Genet.* 2016;17:224−238.
9. Lakich D, et al. Inversions disrupting the factor VIII gene are a common cause of severe haemophilia A. *Nat Genet.* 1993;5:236−241.
10. Puig M, et al. Human inversions and their functional consequences. *Brief Funct Genomics.* 2015;14:369−379.
11. Amendola LM, et al. Performance of ACMG-AMP Variant-interpretation guidelines among nine laboratories in the Clinical Sequencing Exploratory Research Consortium. *Am J Hum Genet.* 2016;99:247.
12. Tryka KA, et al. NCBI's Database of Genotypes and Phenotypes: dbGaP. *Nucleic Acids Res.* 2014;42:D975−D979.
13. Landrum MJ, et al. ClinVar: public archive of interpretations of clinically relevant variants. *Nucleic Acids Res.* 2016;44:D862−D868.
14. Harrison SM, et al. Using ClinVar as a resource to support variant interpretation. *Curr Protoc Hum Genet.* 2016;89: 1−23, 8.16.
15. Fokkema IF, et al. LOVD v.2.0: the next generation in gene variant databases. *Hum Mutat.* 2011;32:557−563.
16. Revy P, et al. The repair of DNA damages/modifications during the maturation of the immune system: lessons from human primary immunodeficiency disorders and animal models. *Adv Immunol.* 2005;87:237−295.
17. Kovanen PE, Leonard WJ. Cytokines and immunodeficiency diseases: critical roles of the gamma(c)-dependent cytokines interleukins 2, 4, 7, 9, 15, and 21, and their signaling pathways. *Immunol Rev.* 2004;202: 67−83.
18. Choi Y, Simon-Stoos K, Puck JM. Hypo-active variant of IL-2 and associated decreased T cell activation contribute to impaired apoptosis in autoimmune prone MRL mice. *Eur J Immunol.* 2002;32:677−685.
19. Diehl AG, Boyle AP. Deciphering ENCODE. *Trends Genet.* 2016;32:238−249.
20. ENCODE Project Consortium. An integrated encyclopedia of DNA elements in the human genome. *Nature.* 2012; 489:57−74.
21. Doolittle WF. Is junk DNA bunk? A critique of ENCODE. *Proc Natl Acad Sci USA.* 2013;110:5294−5300.
22. Eddy SR. The ENCODE project: missteps overshadowing a success. *Curr Biol.* 2013;23:R259−R261.
23. Wijmenga C, Zhernakova. The importance of cohort studies in the post-GWAS era. *Nat Genet.* 2018;50: 322−329.

24. Al-Herz W. Primary immunodeficiency disorders in Kuwait: first report from Kuwait National Primary Immunodeficiency Registry (2004—2006). *J Clin Immunol.* 2008; 28:186—193.

25. Al-Herz W, et al. Parental consanguinity and the risk of primary immunodeficiency disorders: report from the Kuwait National Primary Immunodeficiency Disorders Registry. *Int Arch Allergy Immunol.* 2011;154:76—80.

26. Yang Y, et al. Molecular findings among patients referred for clinical whole-exome sequencing. *JAMA.* 2014;312: 1870—1879.

27. Chan AY, et al. A novel human autoimmune syndrome caused by combined hypomorphic and activating mutations in ZAP-70. *J Exp Med.* 2016;213:155—165.

28. Chong JX, et al. The genetic basis of mendelian phenotypes: discoveries, challenges, and opportunities. *Am J Hum Genet.* 2015;97:199—215.

CHAPTER 2

Principles of Flow Cytometry

THOMAS A. FLEISHER • JOAO B. OLIVEIRA • SERGIO D. ROSENZWEIG

Flow cytometry has become a standard laboratory tool in the evaluation of hematopoietic cells, including the identification of leukocyte populations and subpopulations, a method referred to as *immunophenotyping*. The clinical application of this technology has been facilitated by the development of instruments and data analysis systems suitable for routine use in diagnostic laboratories. In addition, the expanded range of monoclonal antibodies (mAbs) specific for lymphocyte (and other hematopoietic cell) surface antigens directly conjugated to a number of different fluorescent indicators (fluorochromes) provides an extensive panel of reagents that facilitate multicolor (polychromatic) studies.

The clinical needs that pushed this technology date back to the emergence of absolute CD4 T-cell counts as a critical measure for disease assessment and follow-up in managing patients infected with human immunodeficiency virus (HIV). Flow cytometry applied in the monitoring of HIV infection was followed by the routine application of cell characterization by flow cytometry in the evaluation of hematologic malignancies and, more recently, in the study of immunodeficiency disorders and other immune-mediated diseases.

Recent advances in instrumentation and fluorochrome chemistry now allow for routine polychromatic flow cytometry studies, with concomitant assessment of cell surface markers and intracellular parameters, including intracellular proteins, phosphoproteins, and cytokines, as well as identification of changes linked to cellular activation and apoptosis. Intracellular flow cytometry also can be applied to evaluate cell cycle status (*i.e.*, G_0-G_1, S, G_2-M) based on DNA staining, which is useful in evaluating tumor cells and assessing the *in vitro* lymphocyte response to various stimuli. Additionally, evaluation of lymphocyte proliferation can be performed with cell tracking dyes that allow quantitation of the rounds of cell division associated with cell activation, and techniques to assess immune cell–mediated cytotoxicity have also been developed. Finally, characterization of antigen-specific T cells following immunization or associated with normal and/or abnormal immune responses in association with disease states can be accomplished by using multimer technology as well as intracellular cytokine detection following antigen exposure.

This chapter focuses on the basic concepts of flow cytometry, including instrument characteristics, data management, lymphocyte gating, and directed use of test reagents. In addition, it provides a brief overview of intracellular protein detection, cell activation and cell-mediated cytotoxicity studies, cell cycle analysis, apoptosis detection, and multimer technology, focusing on the appropriate application of these approaches as well as their limitations.

INSTRUMENTATION

The basic components of a flow cytometer, as shown in Fig. 2.1, include an illumination source, an optical bench, a fluidic system, electronics, and a computer.[1] Briefly, stained cells flow into single file by the fluidic system and are interrogated by one or more light sources; these sources generate light signals, which are detected by the optical system to the photodetectors, which, in turn, convert light into electronic signals for storage and subsequent analysis. This process is discussed further in the section below.

The fluidic system lies at the heart of the flow cytometer and consists of isotonic sheath fluid that moves the sample stream containing the cells. This is accomplished by injecting the cell sample into flowing sheath fluid, establishing a hydrodynamically focused single-file flow of cells (particles) that move through the analysis point while maintaining the cell stream in a constant, central location.[2] The centrally focused cell stream ensures that the illumination of all cells is virtually equivalent. Thus the difference in magnitude of the emission signal(s) generated from each cell reflects biological differences between the cells (rather than reflecting the variation in the illumination energy if the cells were not tightly focused). The use of hydrodynamic focusing has the additional advantage

Core Laboratory Technologies in Clinical Immunology. https://doi.org/10.1016/B978-0-323-66149-2.00002-5

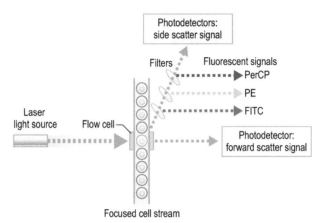

FIG. 2.1 Simplified Design of a Flow Cytometer With Single Illumination Source (Laser) Configuration to Collect Five Parameters. These include the two nonfluorescent parameters (blue light), forward and side scatter, as well as three fluorescent parameters, green (FITC), orange (PE), and red (PerCP) light.

of producing little or no change in cell shape, although it may have an effect on cell orientation. The consistency in maintaining cell shape facilitates distinguishing "architectural" differences between specific leukocyte types (see Gating section).[3] However, this method can generate single-file cell rows with precision only up to a flow rate of 60 to 100 μL/min, which can lead to long acquisition times for the detection of very rare events. To overcome this problem, recently introduced flow cytometry instruments utilize acoustic focusing, which align cells through the use of sound waves, allowing sample flow rates of up to 1000 μL/min, without loss of signal quality.[4,5]

Illumination in standard clinical instruments is generated by two or more lasers, each of which provides a specific monochromatic light source (*e.g.*, a sapphire laser generates a 488-nm-wavelength [blue] beam). Modern lasers are small and available in multiple wavelengths, including ultraviolet (350 nm), violet (405 nm), blue (488 nm), green (532 nm), yellow (560 nm), orange (610 nm), and red (633 nm), permitting the simultaneous use of multiple fluorochromes having different excitation requirements.[6] The point where the light illuminates the cell in analytical instruments occurs within a flow cell, while in cell sorters, the beam intersects cells flowing as a stream in air. The optical bench contains lenses that shape and focus the illumination beam to ensure consistent excitation energy at the analysis point.

The illumination of a cell generates both nonfluorescent and fluorescent signals, which are collected and measured by optically coupling the signal to a detection system consisting of filters, each of which is linked to a photodetector. The filters are chosen to allow the nonfluorescent signals to be measured at the same wavelength as the excitation signal (*e.g.*, 488 nm from a blue light source) for the forward- and side-scatter channels (see Gating section), whereas those for the fluorescence channels utilize specific filters that allow passage of light with wavelengths specific to each fluorescence reagents (*e.g.*, green, orange, or red; see section on fluorescence reagents). The number and arrangement of the photodetectors allows for the simultaneous evaluation of multiple colors (parameters) for each cell, with a report describing a modified clinical instrument capable of evaluating 17 or more colors simultaneously from each cell evaluated.[7]

The internal electronics in the flow cytometer provides the system for converting analog light signals (photoelectrons) received at the photodetectors into digital signals for acquisition and storage in a computer. The intensity of these converted signals is measured on a relative scale that is generally set in either 256 or 1024 equal increments (referred to as *channels*) for display and analysis. A number of specialized analysis programs are available, and results are depicted graphically as single-parameter histograms displaying specific light (fluorescence) intensity (*x*-axis) versus cell number (*y*-axis) (Fig. 2.2), or two-color displays where the *x*-axis and the *y*-axis reflect the light intensity of the two colors, and the cell numbers are represented via dot, pseudocolor, contour, or density plots (Fig. 2.3). Most analysis programs enable the operator to evaluate the number and percentage of events, mean and/or median channel fluorescence, and selected statistical measures for each

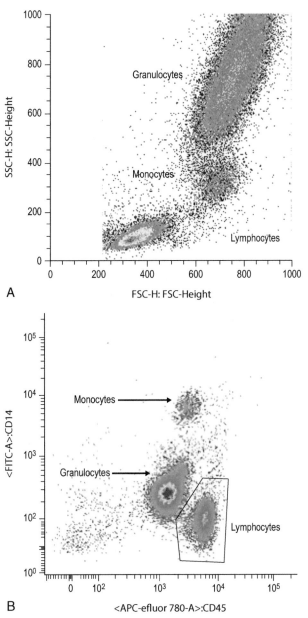

FIG. 2.2 (A) Forward- and side-scatter dot plots on lysed whole blood, demonstrating the basic three-part leukocyte differential with lymphocytes, monocytes, and granulocytes. (B) Dot plot with DC45/CD14 gating reagents showing the fluorescence distribution of all the three leukocyte types identified to include lymphocytes, monocytes, and granulocytes, as well as a small number of nonlysed red blood cells and/or debris.

identified cell, and these can be aggregated into specific populations and/or subpopulations of cells. Thus a flow cytometer provides a platform with the capacity to assess multiple pieces of discrete information (parameters) generated from each individual cell contained within a large number of cells present in the test sample, and these are typically accrued at rates of 1000–2000 (or more) cells per second.

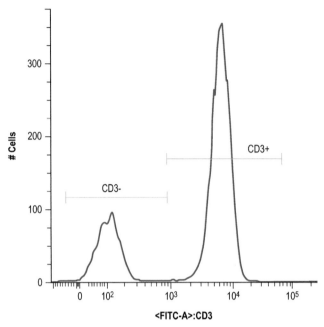

FIG. 2.3 Single-parameter histogram for lymphocyte CD3 expression demonstrating the negative, non—T-cell population (B cells, natural killer [NK] cells), and a positive T-cell population. Integrating the area under each curve would provide the numbers and percentage of cells present in each respective subpopulation.

FLUORESCENCE REAGENTS

Standard mAb reagents for clinical use are typically directly conjugated to a fluorochrome, a dye that absorbs and emits light of different wavelengths based on the energy lost during the return of excited electrons to their ground state associated with illumination by a specific wavelength of light. Thus the emitted light has a longer wavelength (lower energy) than the wavelength of the excitation beam. The number of commercially available fluorochromes has increased dramatically with the routine use of dye conjugates and instruments with three or more lasers.[8] Commonly used fluorochromes in clinical immunophenotyping include the organic dyes fluorescein isothiocyanate (FITC), phycoerythrin (PE), peridin chlorophyll protein (PerCP), and allophycocyanin (APC). Conjugations of PE and APC to cyanines (Cy5, Cy5.5, and Cy7) and Alexa Fluor dyes produce tandem dyes with additional emission spectra, based on energy transfer from one fluorochrome to the second fluorochrome serving as the source of emitted light. This allows for the simultaneous evaluation of 6—8 colors in most current clinical instruments with only two or three lasers.

One recent advance in the field was the development of a new class of inorganic fluorescent semiconductor nanocrystals, named *quantum dots* (QDs).[9] These particles are perfectly suited for polychromatic flow cytometry, as they have broad excitation spectra (525—800 nm) and sharp, discrete emission spectra that varies depending on their core size.[9] This means that QDs of different sizes (and consequently of different colors) can be excited by the same laser source, allowing simpler multiplexing.[9] In addition, QDs have high quantum yield, high molar extinction coefficients, and extraordinary resistance to photodegradation and chemical degradation. These qualities make them perfectly suitable for use in biological studies, including intracellular *in vivo* imaging, fluorescence resonance energy transfer (FRET) analysis, and dynamic imaging of single proteins for longer periods.[9]

Additional dyes are available for functional studies and include calcium-sensitive dyes (*e.g.*, fluo-3), glutathione-sensitive dyes (*e.g.*, monochlorobimane), and hydrogen peroxide (H_2O_2)-responsive dyes (*e.g.*, dihydrorhodamine 123 [DHR123]).[10,11] Assessment of DNA content can be performed with dyes that intercalate double-stranded DNA and RNA, including propidium iodide (PI) and ethidium bromide.[12] In addition, there are ultraviolet-excited dyes that are highly specific for DNA, including Hoechst 33258 and 4,6-diamidino-2-phenylindole (DAPI); acridine orange is used for simultaneous staining of DNA/RNA.[12]

DATA ANALYSIS
Gating

Key Concepts
Gating

- Method for defining cell population of interest
- Typically performed using forward and side scatter as well as lineage-specific antibodies

The proper assessment of specific cell types within a mixture requires initial identification of lineage-specific cells, an approach referred to as *gating*. In practical terms, immunophenotyping focused on lymphocytes requires minimizing the nonlymphocytes included in the evaluation, and this is accomplished by lymphocyte gating. The standard sample for clinical studies is anticoagulated whole blood; directing the study to lymphocytes requires eliminating the great majority of nonlymphocytes from the collected data such that the expression of a percentage for a specific cell subpopulation is an accurate measurement. Without gating, data can also be negatively impacted by coexpression of surface antigens on different cell lineages (*e.g.*, CD4 is found on lymphocytes and monocytes at varying densities). In addition, nonspecific binding of monoclonal reagents through Fcγ receptors, and the level of cytophilic human immunoglobulin (Ig), varies between cell types, making appropriate gating crucial to generate valid data. These techniques are also used to focus the evaluation on other hematopoietic cells, including monocytes, granulocytes, eosinophils, erythrocytes, and platelets.

Initial gating to focus on a specific leukocyte population typically involves the use of two nonfluorescent parameters, forward scatter (FSC) and side scatter (SSC) (see Fig. 2.2A).[3] FSC is a reflection of cellular cross-sectional area (direct relationship to cell size), whereas SSC is an indication of the cellular granularity. The combination of these two nonfluorescent parameters provides a three-part differential in red blood cell (RBC)-lysed whole blood that distinguishes between normal lymphocytes, monocytes, and granulocytes. As seen in Fig. 2.2A, among leukocytes, lymphocytes have the lowest FSC and SSC, monocytes have higher FSC and SSC, and granulocytes have the greatest SSC. This method is effective in distinguishing a relatively pure population of lymphocytes under most circumstances. However, the presence of nucleated RBCs, large platelets, increased basophils, or other particulate debris can produce contaminating events (cells) within this "lymphocyte gate." Furthermore, malignant or activated lymphoid cells may not fit into the previously outlined standard light scatter patterns.

A method for confirming the integrity of the light scatter–based lymphocyte gate uses the directly conjugated monoclonal "gating" reagents, anti-CD45 and anti-CD14.[13] These two mAbs more accurately identify the three-part differential. Lymphocytes have the highest level of CD45 binding but are negative for CD14; granulocytes have a lower level of CD45 binding and an intermediate level of CD14 expression; and monocytes have high levels of both CD45 and CD14 expression (see Fig. 2.2B). Importantly, nonleukocytes, including erythrocytes and platelets, are negative for these markers. However, malignant leukocytes that have characteristics of early precursor cells often have altered CD45 and/or CD14 expression, which must be recognized when studying hematological malignancies. Gating reagents provide a reliable means of checking the light scatter–based lymphocyte gate for the frequency of nonlymphocytes within the gate, as well as the extent of lymphocyte exclusion from the gate. Guidelines for an acceptable degree of contamination within the lymphocyte gate, as well as the level of lymphocyte exclusion, are contained in the US Clinical and Laboratory Standards Institute guideline for lymphocyte immunophenotyping.[14] With the expanded use of polychromatic flow cytometry, some centers now include anti-CD45 in every tube to refine the gate and prevent cell contamination as described above.

Data Display

Key Concepts
Data Presentation

- Fluorescence intensity is plotted versus cell number.
- Flow cytometry can present cumulative data on more than one parameter for each cell.
- Multicolor data presentation can increase cell subpopulation resolution.

The simplest method for demonstrating flow cytometry data is the single-parameter histogram (see Fig. 2.2), a graphic presentation of cell number on the *y*-axis versus fluorescence (light) intensity from a single fluorochrome on the *x*-axis. Integration of curve areas provides the number of cells, and often there are two distinct distributions, one referred to as *negative* identifying cells that are not bound specifically by the monoclonal reagent, and the second represents cells bound by the antibody. Negative distribution actually reflects low-level fluorescence resulting from cellular autofluorescence together with any nonspecific binding of the monoclonal reagent(s), and the magnitude of both phenomena varies among different cell types. Interpretation of data is simplified when there are two distinct cell populations (*i.e.*, negative and positive), while the evaluation of two overlapping distributions is more difficult.

Multiparameter data can be evaluated by using a series of single-parameter histograms that consider each fluorochrome independently. However, it is more informative to present two parameters simultaneously by using a correlated display (Fig. 2.4), and two-color displays are recommended for clinical flow cytometry.[15] This approach enables the simultaneous visualization of four different populations: A^+/B^-, A^-/B^+, A^+/B^+, and A^-/B^-. More recently, these displays were developed further to include a mixture of logarithmic (for higher intensity expression) and linear (for lower intensity expression) intensity for each axis to allow for better interpretation of events with very low, zero, or negative fluorescence. This combined-display approach resolves the previous problem of a large number of events being displayed compacted against the axes, even with properly compensated samples, and will be used in the illustrations throughout this chapter.[16]

The simultaneous use of n monoclonal reagents can identify a total of 2^n subpopulations. These different subsets can be identified sequentially by first dividing the cells into those that are positive versus those that are negative with one reagent and then evaluating the defined subpopulations for the remaining two reagents using a two-color approach. Alternatively, more modern software can represent multiple populations as polychromatic plots, which

can simplify data analysis.[17] The polychromatic approach can provide a means to further resolve subpopulations and has been particularly useful in the evaluation of cellular differentiation, activation, and functional correlates, as well as clarifying overlapping cell subpopulations.

Positive-Negative Discrimination

The evaluation of clinical immunophenotyping data requires establishing criteria for the boundaries between negative or nonstained (autofluorescence plus nonspecifically stained) cells and positive (specifically stained) cells. A commonly used approach involves using directly conjugated control mAbs of the appropriate class or subclass (*e.g.*, IgG1, IgG2a, IgG2b, or IgM) that do not specifically react with human lymphocyte surface antigens (commonly referred to as "isotype controls"). The marker (discriminator) is set at the fluorescence histogram channel number such that it includes 98–99% of the negative cells (Fig. 2.5A).

As previously noted, *negative* refers to the aggregate of baseline cellular autofluorescence plus nonspecific reagent binding, and this can vary according to the cell type. For this reason, the use of isotype controls may not correctly identify the positive-negative threshold for specific cell types, particularly when staining dimly expressed proteins. Additionally, to perfectly mimic the specific antibody used, the isotype control would need to have the same antibody to fluorochrome ratio and brightness, something that is not easily accomplished. To overcome these difficulties, an alternative method for positive-negative discrimination, fluorescence-minus-one (FMO), has been developed.[18]

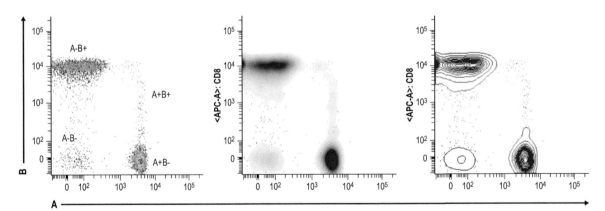

FIG. 2.4 Dot Pseudocolor *(Left)*, Density *(Middle)*, and Contour *(Right)* Displays Based on the Same Two-Color Parameter Data. All three techniques enable simultaneous evaluation of both parameters, in this case evaluating the expression of markers A and B. These plots identify four populations of cells, those expressing only A or B, those expressing both A and B (very few), and those expressing neither A nor B.

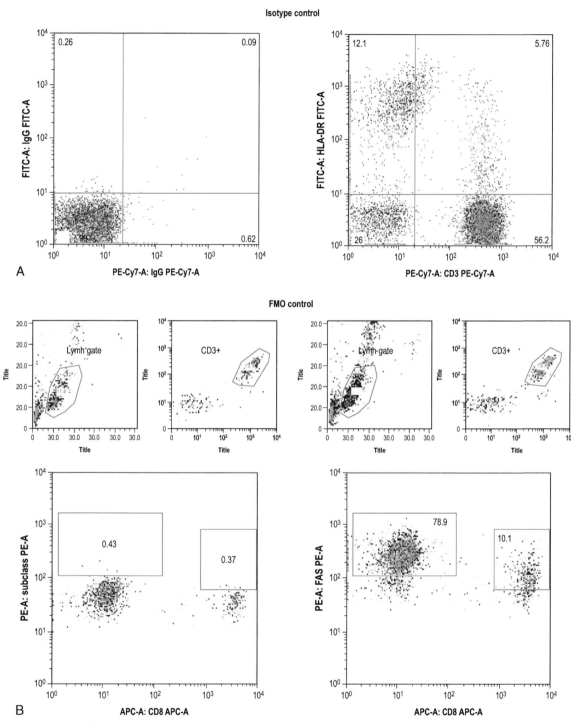

FIG. 2.5 Strategies for Positive-Negative Discrimination. (A) Nonspecific antibodies (isotypes) were used to stain the sample shown on the left and the positivity threshold determined and applied to the sample on the right. (B) Fluorescence-minus-one (FMO). The positivity threshold was determined by staining the sample on the left with the population-specific markers (CD3, TCRαβ, and CD8) and omitting FAS. The panel on the right contains FAS. Note that the positivity threshold is slightly different for CD8$^+$ and CD8$^-$ cells.

FMO involves the staining of the sample with all the antibodies of interest, except the one targeted for positive-negative threshold. As an example, to define the negative threshold for the protein FAS (CD95) in $CD8^+$ and $CD8^-$ T cells, the FMO control tube would include the cell subset–specific markers (CD3, TCRαβ, and CD8) and omit anti-FAS. After appropriate gating on that population, the threshold can be adequately defined, and it is different for the two exemplified populations (see Fig. 2.5B, *right panel*). One obvious limitation of this method is the higher cost, given that multiple control tubes need to be set up for each sample.

Compensation

The fluorescence signals emitted by different fluorochromes are not completely separated by the filters. This can lead to signal overlap, which is corrected by electronic subtraction of the overlapping signal, a process referred to as *compensation*. The overlap is particularly significant when using multiple fluorochromes, each with different spectral properties.[18] The compensation process involves subtraction of the "spillover" signal detected by the photodetector generated by samples stained with only one fluorochrome. Currently, most flow cytometry analysis software products allow for off-line compensation, where the single reagent stained tubes are used to create a compensation matrix, which is then applied to all the tubes in the experiment. This allows for much simplified compensation procedures, without the need for any hardware compensation during data collection.

Quality Control

Quality control is a critical component of clinical flow cytometry to ensure optimal results.[19] This includes monitoring instrument setup and performance, optimizing sample preparation and reagents, and standardizing controls and data interpretation. Quantitative flow cytometry based on a fluorescence standard curve provides quantitative data in units referred to as *molecular equivalents of soluble fluorochrome* (MESF). When properly constructed standard curves are used, quantitative data for different reagents can be generated and compared. Finally, participation in interlaboratory proficiency testing surveys, such as the triannual samples provided by the College of American Pathologists (CAP), is an important additional measure to monitor laboratory performance, and this is mandated in US clinical laboratories by the Clinical Laboratory Improvement Amendment of 1988 (CLIA 88).

Methods

Whole-blood lysis represents the most common technique used for sample preparation and consists of mixing a fixed volume of anticoagulated whole blood (or bone marrow) with one or more directly conjugated mAbs, followed by incubation at a designated temperature and time.[20] Next, RBCs are lysed, and the sample is washed and then run into the flow cytometer, usually following fixation in paraformaldehyde to reduce the risk of infection. Nonlysed cells that remain include all peripheral blood leukocytes as well as any nonlysed RBCs, platelets, and debris. The heterogeneity of the sample necessitates careful lymphocyte gating (see Gating section above) to generate accurate immunophenotyping data. The advantages of the whole-blood-lysis method include fewer preparation steps, less sample handling, and a lower likelihood of differential lymphocyte loss that can occur when density gradient techniques are used to prepare mononuclear cells for analysis. Alternative sources of cells (*e.g.,* bone marrow, bronchial alveolar lavage fluid, fine-needle aspirates) can also be evaluated with flow cytometry.[21] Patient studies must be determined with the same methods and reagents as used in the determination of the control ranges to ensure comparability. The number of events (cells) analyzed typically ranges from 10 000 to 20 000 in routine clinical studies but must be increased when evaluating very small subpopulations of cells to produce statistically relevant data necessary in rare-event analysis.

The application of control ranges must take into account the fact that significant changes take place in lymphocyte distribution and development during childhood, as well as changes in lymphocytes that occur among the very old.[22,23] In addition, since immunophenotypic differences can be induced by drugs, including tobacco products, information on current medications should be obtained, whenever possible. Other factors can also have an impact on lymphocyte distribution, including race, gender, diurnal variation, and recent or intercurrent infections.[24]

The choice of immunophenotyping reagents depends on the cells being targeted for study and the question being asked. However, regardless of the specific setup, the inclusion of a tube with gating reagents (anti-CD45 and anti-CD14) to confirm the integrity of the standard lymphocyte gate is recommended.[13] In addition, control reagents should be included to establish the fluorescence intensity of negative (unstained) cells. Important internal controls include a pan-T-, B-, and natural killer (NK)-cell marker for every sample (Table 2.1), based on the principle that the whole is

TABLE 2.1
Selected Lymphocyte Surface Molecules for Immunophenotyping

T CELLS

Pan-T cell: CD3, CD2, CD7, CD5
Major T-cell subset: CD4, CD8
Surface antigens associated with function: CD28, CD31, CD38, CD45RA, CD45RO, CD62L, CXCR7
Activation antigens: CD25, CD40L, CD69, CD71, HLA-DR

B CELLS

Pan-B cell: CD19, CD20, surface immunoglobulin
Major B-cell subset: CD5, CD21
Surface antigens associated with function: CD27, CD40, CD80, CD86
Activation antigens: CD23, CD25

NK CELLS

Pan-natural killer (NK) cell: CD16, CD56
NK subset: CD2, CD8, CD57

biological findings may also be uncovered through this type of evaluation (e.g., the presence of an increased population of $CD4^-/CD8^-$ double-negative T cells).[25]

The challenge in performing immunophenotyping is to accurately identify cells with specific surface characteristics (antigens). As previously noted, the capacity to discriminate cell subpopulations is often enhanced through the directed use of antibody combinations. The typical data generated consist of the percentage of negative versus positive cells when using one reagent and multiple subpopulations when using more than one reagent. Regardless of the experimental design, it is important to consider not only the percentage of cells within each subpopulation but also the absolute number of cells. This is most commonly obtained by multiplying the relevant percentage from the flow cytometer by the absolute lymphocyte count obtained by using a white blood cell (WBC) count and differential. For example, when assaying for CD4 T-cell counts, the percentage of $CD4^+$ cells is multiplied by the peripheral absolute lymphocyte count to yield the absolute CD4 count. A potential problem with this approach is the requirement for two separate procedures (i.e., dual platforms) to generate the final result. This introduces the possibility of additive error, based on the inherent errors of the two different methods. It also has fueled a search for approaches that facilitate performing both tasks by flow cytometry (i.e., a single platform). One alternative involves the inclusion of a fixed number of fluorescent beads (in a defined volume) in each tube as a reference standard to generate absolute numbers without requiring the use of the complete blood count (CBC) and differential to generate a lymphocyte count. An alternative approach involves the use of impedance-based cell counting in the flow cytometer to generate an absolute lymphocyte count (dependent on a fixed volume of sample being run) and then generating both percentage and absolute number of cells in each specific population or subpopulation. Regardless of the approach, the reporting of both percentages and absolute numbers is necessary when immunophenotyping peripheral lymphocytes.

The objective of evaluating malignant cells is often to characterize the lineage and differentiation level of the abnormal cells, rather than quantifying subpopulations. The pattern of reactivity combined with fluorescence intensity is often useful in identifying leukemic patterns, whereas the absolute number of cells usually is not required. However, flow-cytometric detection and quantitation of rare abnormal cells can be useful in evaluating for minimal residual disease after therapy in lymphoproliferative disorders.

the sum of its parts. Thus the total percentage of lymphocytes in the gate determined by the gating reagents should approximately equal the sum of the percentages for T, B, and NK cells. A technical or biological explanation must be identified when this relationship does not hold. Biological explanations for a significant difference would include the presence of immature or malignant cells that were not identified by standard pan-T-, B-, and NK-cell reagents. Also, if the gating reagents (CD45/CD14) had not been included, contaminating cells (e.g., myeloid precursors, nucleated RBCs, large platelets) with FSC and SSC characteristics similar to those of lymphocytes could not be ruled out. Potential technical problems include reagent or fluorochrome degradation, failure to add a reagent, and a host of others. Evidence for any major technical error should result in repeating the study.

Additional data that can be used for controls depend on the setup. For example, the availability of multiple antibodies that identify a similar cell subpopulation can serve as a useful check (e.g., total T cells by comparing CD3 and CD5 or CD2; total B cells by comparing CD19 and CD20). In addition, the use of specific reagents in >1 tube enables comparison between the repeat values as a measure of consistency. The application of internal checks should be performed by the flow operator as a simple means of confirming the validity of the data. Insights regarding unusual

PRACTICAL APPLICATIONS OF FLOW CYTOMETRY
Immunophenotyping Studies

> **Clinical Relevance**
> *Immunophenotyping Studies*
>
> - Immunotyping studies can be used to identify cell subsets, lineage, stage of cell differentiation, state of cell activation, and clonality.
> - Lymphocyte results should be checked with T cells + B cells + natural killer (NK) cells = ~100%.
> - Immunophenotyping studies are not the equivalent of lymphocyte function studies.

Most immunophenotyping studies aim to enumerate specific cell subpopulations, evaluate for the presence or absence of particular surface antigens, identify the differentiation level of specific cells, determine cell lineage, evaluate for functional correlates based on specific antigen expression, examine evidence of cell activation, and/or establish evidence of monoclonality.

Quantification of a particular cell subpopulation can be readily accomplished by flow cytometry together with a WBC count and cell differential. The absolute lymphocyte count is used to generate population or subpopulation cell numbers based on the percentages of the respective cell types generated with the flow cytometer. The evaluation of absolute CD4 T-cell counts has formed the basis for monitoring patients with HIV infection.[26] The quantitation of CD34$^+$ hematopoietic stem cells (HSCs) in donor peripheral blood or bone marrow is used in many cellular reconstitution protocols.[27] Subpopulation characterization can also be useful in the evaluation of patients with clinical history and laboratory findings suggestive of immune deficiency.[28,29] This has taken on a higher level of significance in the setting of newborn screening for severe T-cell immune deficiency via the T-cell receptor excision circle (TREC) assay, which, when abnormal, is typically followed by immunophenotyping to evaluate for naïve T cells based on CD45RA, CD127, or CD62L expression.

When evaluating for the presence or absence of surface proteins associated with specific functional attributes, it is important to realize that this approach does not assess the actual functional status of cells. This point is clearly illustrated by the finding of normal B-cell numbers in most patients with common variable immune deficiency despite the fact that these patients fail to produce Igs normally.[30] However, changes in the characteristics of the B cells, particularly relative to memory B cells, provide potential insight into different phenotypes of this disorder and provide additional support for heterogeneity of patients with the disease.[31,32] Because of the limitations of immunophenotyping, when evaluating the status of the immune system, it is common practice to perform cell function testing in parallel.

Flow cytometry can be used to test for the presence or absence of a specific cell surface antigen. An example of this type of application is in the evaluation of a patient with a history of recurrent skin infections, delayed wound healing, and persistent granulocytosis, which suggests a diagnosis of leukocyte adhesion deficiency type 1 (LAD-1).[28,33] This disorder results from a defect in the gene encoding CD18, preventing/decreasing the expression of three different heterodimeric adhesion molecules (β_2 integrins) each containing CD18. This disorder can usually be diagnosed by studying granulocytes (and lymphocytes) for the expression of CD18 (as well as the three isoforms of CD11). Patients often have decreased rather than absent CD18 expression and confirmation of the diagnosis can be accomplished by demonstrating failure of CD18 (and CD11a, CD11b, CD11c) upregulation following granulocyte activation.[28,29]

Immunophenotyping can also help address questions regarding the level of cell differentiation. Antibodies specific to proteins expressed by early (precursor) cells represent one approach and would include evaluating for the thymocyte marker CD1 or the pre-B-cell marker CD10 (CALLA), to cite a few. However, defining the developmental level of a particular cell population or subpopulation is best accomplished by using a panel of reagents that span the natural history of the cell lineage. This approach represents the standard for testing leukemias and lymphomas, which may provide useful prognostic information.[34] In addition to defining the presence or absence of specific antigens, evaluating their level of expression is also valuable, which may be altered in abnormal cells. Malignant cells may also express antigens associated with different lineages and have altered FSC and SSC characteristics, as well as diminished or absent CD45 expression, requiring modified gating approaches.

Issues of monoclonality can be dealt with by using flow cytometry when analyzing B cells and, in some circumstances, when studying T cells. Normally, B cells are a heterogeneous mixture of mutually exclusive κ or λ light-chain-positive cells. Measuring the distribution of κ or λ light-chain-expressing B cells or plasmocytes can be informative with respect to the presence or absence of monoclonality.[35] The capacity to evaluate T-cell monoclonality by flow cytometry is less definitive and consists of using T-cell antigen receptor β-variable

(Vβ) chain-specific reagents looking for evidence of significant overrepresentation of one Vβ chain family. This approach currently consists of setting up a series of tubes, each with three different Vβ family–specific mAbs, one conjugated with FITC, one with PE, and the third with FITC plus PE. This combination enables distinguishing the frequency of each of the three different Vβ families per tube (green+, orange+, green+/orange+) and represents a flow-cytometric method to complement polymerase chain reaction (PCR)-based spectratyping.[36]

The state of lymphocyte activation can be addressed by evaluating for the presence of surface antigens that are found only on activated cells or are upregulated following activation. These include receptors for specific growth factors (*e.g.*, interleukin-2 [IL-2] receptor α chain, CD25), receptors for critical elements required for cell growth (*e.g.*, transferrin receptor, CD71), ligands for cell-cell communication following activation (CD40 ligand [CD152] on activated CD4 T cells), and surface antigens that are upregulated as a result of activation (*e.g.*, adhesion molecules, HLA-DR, CD69). In addition, the memory status of both T cells and B cells can be assessed on the basis of differential surface molecule expression associated with prior antigen encounter. This enables a distinction to be made between naïve T cells that express CD45RA, CD31 (recent thymic emigrants), CD62L, and CXCR7 and memory T cells that express the alternative CD45 isoform, CD45RO (and varied CD62L, or CXCR7, depending on whether the cells are central or effector memory cells).[37] In addition, memory B cells can be detected by the expression of CD27 and can be further divided into isotype-switched and isotype-nonswitched memory cells on the basis of their pattern of surface immunoglobulin expression.[30,38]

Defects associated with familial lymphohistiocytosis (FLH) are generally associated with abnormal NK cell function. Many of the FHL-causing defects can be determined by flow cytometry. For example, signaling lymphocyte activation molecule (SLAM)-associated protein (SAP) and X-linked inhibitor of apoptosis (XIAP) intracellular staining can be used to evaluate for X-linked lymphoproliferative (XLP) disorder types 1 and 2, respectively. Likewise, lack of intracellular perforin expression in NK cells would be indicative of FHL type 2. Additionally, the evaluation of CD107a surface expression, which is normally expressed on cytoplasmic granules and upon incubation with specific target cells (*e.g.*, K562 cells) gets expressed on the surface of NK cells, is useful in determining the underlying genetic defect causing FHL.[39,40] Specifically, lack of CD107a upregulation is suggestive of syntaxin-11 or MUNC-13.4 defects.

INTRACELLULAR EVALUATION
Cellular Activation

> **Clinical Relevance**
> *Intracellular Flow Cytometry*
>
> - Activation-directed studies:
>   - Calcium flux
>   - Intracellular protein phosphorylation
>   - Oxidative burst: neutrophils
> - Intracellular cytokine studies:
>   - Clarify the T-helper-1 (Th1)/Th2/Th17 status of an immune response
>   - Can be assessed in an *in vitro* antigen–specific response
>   - Can be combined with evaluation of cell surface studies

Ligand binding and transmembrane signal transduction resulting in cellular activation can be evaluated by using flow cytometry. Changes in intracellular ionic calcium concentration (Ca^{2+}) can be used to monitor cell activation after ligand binding. These changes are associated with the activation of phospholipase C and protein kinase C. In general, three reagents have been used to measure Ca^{2+}: quin 2, indo-1, and fluo-3. Quin 2 has a low excitation coefficient and is not useful for flow cytometry; indo-1 requires ultraviolet excitation; fluo-3 can be excited by 488 nm but does not permit ratiometric analysis. Nevertheless, because of its ease of use, fluo-3 is currently the most widely used probe for intracytoplasmic Ca^{2+} evaluation by flow cytometry. Strict attention must be paid to loading conditions, the presence or absence of free Ca^{2+} in the medium, experimental temperature, baseline measurements, and calibration. This approach can be combined with cell surface marker or cell cycle evaluation.[10]

Intracellular pH changes related to cellular activation also can be evaluated. The most useful probe for pH is SNARF-1.[10] This probe can be excited at 488 nm and allows for ratiometric analysis with detection wavelengths set for 575 and 640 nm. Glutathione (glutamylcysteinylglycine [GSH]), an important antioxidant generated during cell activation, can be measured by using flow cytometry.[10] The fluorescent probe monochlorobimane is commonly used for this measurement, but it is complicated by the need to determine GSH by an independent method, such as high-performance liquid chromatography (HPLC).

Additional approaches for evaluation of cellular activation include assessment of intranuclear markers

(Ki-67, PCNA) as well as surface proteins that are upregulated following cellular activation (*e.g.*, CD69, CD25, CD71).[41] Actual cell division can be evaluated by using lipophilic membrane dyes (*e.g.*, PKH26, CFSE, Cell Trace Violet), also referred to as *cell tracking dyes*, which lose 50% of their fluorescence with each round of cell division.[42] This approach has become more common in the clinical assessment of lymphocyte function because of the capacity to evaluate specific lymphocyte subpopulations responding to mitogenic and antigenic stimuli. Lipophilic membrane dyes also can be used to label target cells in cell-based cytotoxicity assays.[43] Recently, an approach to evaluate lymphocyte proliferation following cell stimulation has been described by using the modified nucleoside EdU. Detection of DNA synthesis induced by the different activating agents is measured using a copper-catalyzed click chemistry, which results in EdU being covalently bound to a fluorescent azide.[44] This approach allows for assessment of cell proliferation at the cell population or subpopulation (*e.g.*, CD3, CD4, CD8) level and can be used in association with mitogen and recall-antigen stimulation.

Functional evaluation of cell activation can be accomplished with flow cytometry–directed detection of the generation of phosphorylated intracellular proteins associated with specific activation signals. An example of this is the detection of phosphorylated signal transducer and activator of transcription 1 (STAT1) following interferon-γ (IFN-γ) stimulation of monocytes, which has been found to be equal to or more sensitive than immunoblotting.[45] This type of assay requires fixation and permeabilization to allow entry of the specific reagent and now has been extended to a number of additional intracellular proteins that are phosphorylated following exposure of selected cells to specific stimuli. Currently, a number of intracellular signaling proteins that undergo phosphorylation following a specific activation signal can be assessed with flow cytometry by using commercially available reagents, some of which are offered in kit form.

The assessment of oxidative burst following cell stimulation plays a central role in neutrophil function testing where the hydrogen peroxide-sensitive dye DHR123 is used. This procedure involves loading granulocytes with the dye, stimulating with phorbol myristate acetate (PMA), and evaluating for increased fluorescence with flow cytometry.[11,46] This test has proven to be extremely accurate in diagnosing patients with chronic granulomatous disease (CGD) and carriers of X-linked CGD.[46] A major advantage is its sensitivity, which allows for detection of one normal cell in a population of 1000 abnormal cells. This makes assessment

of oxidative burst a useful tool in monitoring allogeneic granulocyte survival after transfusion into patients with CGD, as well as a means of following donor chimerism in the setting of allogeneic stem cell transplantation. It also provides a method to identify corrected cells following gene therapy in CGD and has utility in predicting disease outcome.[47,48]

Intracellular Cytokine Detection

Flow cytometry affords a platform to evaluate cytokine production at the single-cell level by using cytokine-specific, directly conjugated mAbs after fixation and permeabilization of cells.[49] This approach allows for simultaneous detection of two or more intracellular cytokines in combination with cell surface markers or other intracellular markers. Important aspects of intracellular cytokine detection include use of a protein transport inhibitor during activation, use of proper controls, and choice of antibodies. As there is little or no spontaneous cytokine production in circulating human lymphocytes, intracellular cytokine detection requires *in vitro* activation. Initial experience was based on supraphysiological stimulation with use of PMA and ionomycin, but antigen-specific activation systems have also proven to be feasible. It should be emphasized that regardless of the activation method, the duration of activation is an important variable, as individual cells reach maximum cytokine production at different times. In addition, different cytokines have different optimal periods of activation. It is recommended that a proper kinetic profile be established for the biological system or clinical condition being studied.[49]

To increase the amount of intracellular cytokines, inhibitors of intracellular protein transport (*e.g.*, monensin or brefeldin) are commonly used, which leads to accumulation of proteins within the cell. Nonspecific binding of antibody reagents is an issue, as permeabilization allows access not only to the cytokine of interest but also to other proteins present in much greater quantities within the cell than on the cell surface. In addition, fixation further increases nonspecific binding, and use of a negative-control sample, which contains an excess of unlabeled or "cold" anticytokine antibody, as well as a subclass-matched or FMO-control sample provides optimal control. When the conjugated anticytokine is added to the negative-control sample, it can only bind to other proteins in a nonspecific manner, thereby providing a measure to discriminate between specific and nonspecific binding. The use of directly conjugated anticytokine antibodies not only simplifies the staining procedure but also provides the best distinction between specific and nonspecific binding. Because the fixation agent may change the native state of certain epitopes, it is also important to use antibodies that recognize antigens after fixation when combining cell surface characterization with intracellular cytokine evaluation.

One of the main applications of intracellular cytokine detection by flow cytometry has been the study and refinement of the T-helper (Th)1/Th2/Th17 paradigms. It has recently become clear that the regulated secretion of cytokines can be used to study the response of individual T cells to both polyclonal stimuli and specific antigens. Measuring antigen-specific T-cell cytokine expression in response to specific antigen offers a useful alternative to the multimer-based approach (discussed below) to quantify the frequency of antigen-specific T cells.[50]

Cell Cycle Analysis

> **Clinical Relevance**
> *Cell Cycle Analysis*
>
> - Useful for screening percentage of S phase and aneuploidy
> - Can be combined with cell surface studies
> - Can be combined with markers of apoptosis

In addition to surface immunophenotyping and cytoplasmic characterization, flow cytometry is also used in cell cycle analysis. PI is the most commonly used fluorochrome because of its optimal linear DNA-binding capacity in a variety of different cell types. Thus a single-parameter histogram of DNA content using PI readily permits the determination of cell cycle compartments, expressed as the percentage of cells in $G_0–G_1$, S, and $G_2–M$ (Fig. 2.6A). In addition to these conventional parameters, the presence or absence of aneuploidy can be determined by inspection of the $G_0–G_1$ peak and/or use of a DNA index (ratio of abnormal DNA content to a diploid DNA standard). Also, elevation in the S and/or $G_2–M$ phase can be detected. The optimal display of these data uses a combination of SSC versus DNA content. Cells observed on the histogram in the area below the level of $G_0–G_1$ may be undergoing apoptosis.[51] When dealing with DNA staining, a consistent cellular source of DNA (*e.g.,* chicken erythrocytes) should be used as an internal reference for evaluating DNA content and evaluating the cell cycle distribution.

It should be noted that several different computer algorithms have been developed to determine the relative proportion of each cell cycle compartment, and the selection of a software program is not a trivial process. The major instrument manufacturers supply cell cycle analysis programs, and third-party programs are also available. Generally, the optimal program should be capable of modeling two or more aneuploid populations, subtracting debris (particularly if formalin-fixed, paraffin-embedded [FFPE] archival material is used) and accurately estimating S-phase cells.[51,52] The combination of a surface marker and the cell cycle has been very useful in differentiating normal cell populations from tumor cell populations. One example is the use of anti-κ-, anti-λ-, or B-cell reagents to separate the aneuploid B-cell clone from the remaining normal, reactive B cells in a lymphoid cell mixture. Another uses cytokeratin as a marker to distinguish between tumor cells and inflammatory cells.

The other major event that has occurred in cell cycle analysis has been the development of technology using the incorporation of bromodeoxyuridine.[53] This thymidine analogue is used to directly determine the

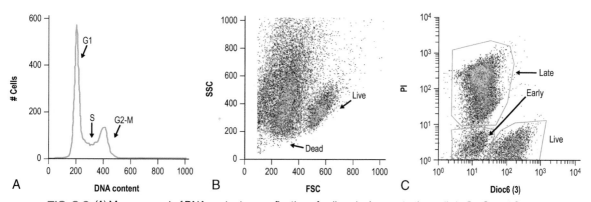

FIG. 2.6 (A) Measurement of DNA content as a reflection of cell cycle demonstrating cells in G_1, S, and $G_2–M$ phases. (B) Evaluation of live versus dead cells based on forward-(FSC) and side-scatter (SSC) characteristics. (C) Determination of cell apoptosis using propidium iodide (PI) and Dioc6 (3) identifying cells that recently initiated apoptosis (early), cells that are dead (late), and cells that are alive (live).

percentage of S-phase cells. Additionally, when used in kinetic studies, it permits determination of individual times for the components of the cell cycle and determination of the growth fraction. Finally, recent developments have resulted in the availability of two anticyclin reagents to evaluate cell cycle transition points in malignant cells.[54]

APOPTOSIS DETECTION

Flow cytometry has become the method of choice for the detection and quantification of cellular apoptosis[55] in part because of its capacity for rapid assessment of a large number of cells and samples. Many distinct features of an apoptotic cell can be evaluated by using flow cytometry based on light scatter, plasma membrane changes, mitochondrial transmembrane potential, DNA content, and DNA integrity.

The light scattering properties of a cell undergoing programmed cell death are the simplest attributes that can be assessed by flow cytometry. Dying cells typically shrink, producing a loss in FSC, and, despite an initial transient increase in SSC, ultimately demonstrate a decrease in SSC (see Fig. 2.6B). The use of light scatter can be combined with cell surface staining to help characterize the dying cells. However, scatter changes alone are not specific to apoptosis and should be accompanied by an additional characteristic associated with cell death. Live cells have phospholipids asymmetrically distributed in inner and outer plasma membranes, with phosphatidylcholine and sphingomyelin on the outer surface and phosphatidylserine (PS) on the inner side. Early during apoptosis cells lose asymmetry, exposing PS on the outside. Annexin V is a protein that binds preferentially to negatively charged phospholipids, such as PS, and directly conjugated annexin V is a useful reagent for the specific detection of apoptotic cells.[55]

Another characteristic of plasma membranes associated with live cells is that they exclude charged cationic dyes, such as PI and 7-amino-actinomycin-D (7-AAD). Consequently, only cells in a late stage of apoptosis, with ruptured cell membranes, will take up these dyes. Thus the combined use of cationic dyes (*e.g.*, PI) with annexin V allows for discrimination between live cells (annexin V negative/ PI negative), early apoptotic cells (annexin V positive/ PI negative), and late apoptotic cells (annexin V positive/ PI positive).

Assessment of mitochondrial transmembrane potential ($\Delta\psi$m) is yet another technique used to identify apoptotic cells. Cells decrease $\Delta\psi$m very early in the apoptotic process, before rupture of the plasma membrane, losing the ability to accumulate potential-dependent dyes, such as rhodamine 123, JC-1, or 3,3′-dihexyloxacarbocyanine iodide (Dioc6^3). These dyes can also be used with PI to detect cells in the different stages of apoptosis (see Fig. 2.6C).

Measurement of DNA content can also be employed to distinguish live cells from dead cells, as described above (see Cell Cycle Analysis section). This kind of analysis has to be done by using a linear scale, not a logarithmic scale, to discriminate dying cells from debris. DNA cleavage also exposes −OH termini associated with the DNA breaks, and these can be detected via the attachment of fluorochrome-conjugated deoxynucleotides, in a reaction catalyzed by exogenous TdT, a technique called *TUNEL.*

PEPTIDE-MHC MULTIMERS

> **Key Concepts**
> *Peptide-MHC Tetramers*
>
> - Useful for assessing the number of antigen-specific T cells
> - Can be directed at both CD4$^+$ and CD8$^+$ T cells
> - Requires information about the antigenic peptide and human leukocyte antigen (HLA) (major histocompatibility complex [MHC]) restriction

In contrast to B cells, direct visualization of antigen-specific T cells *ex vivo* has, until recently, been unsuccessful. In 1996, Altman et al. introduced a novel flow cytometry–based methodology that enables the direct visualization and quantification of antigen-specific T cells.[56] Soluble peptide-MHC multimers are generated such that multiple T-cell receptors (TCRs) are engaged at the same time, which means that the avidity of these multimeric ligands for the peptide-specific TCR is greatly increased. The methodology involves engineering a biotinylation recognition sequence on the −COOH terminus of the extracellular domain of one chain of the MHC molecule, which, after combining with a specific antigenic peptide, is bound by avidin or streptavidin. As both avidin and streptavidin have four biotin-binding sites, the result is a tetrameric peptide-MHC complex that serves as a ligand for T cells specific for both the peptide and the MHC.

Flow-cytometric detection is achieved by labeling streptavidin with a fluorochrome. The major pitfall of this approach is the need to know the antigen-derived peptide and its HLA restrictions, as well as the HLA type of each subject studied. Since the initial report, an increasing number of tetramer-based studies have been performed. Most have focused on the MHC class I–mediated immune response, in both mice and humans, to a variety of infectious agents, including cytomegalovirus (CMV), HIV, Epstein-Barr virus (EBV), and others. Since the initial description with class I–restricted recognition, detection of antigen-specific CD4 T cells with tetramers of soluble MHC class II molecules and covalently linked peptide has also been reported.[57]

In addition to demonstrating the feasibility of this approach, published studies have provided several new insights into the MHC class I–mediated immune response. For example, it has become clear that the extent of the MHC class I–mediated cellular response is much greater than previously estimated. Furthermore, the extensive proliferation of CD8 T cells during an acute infection is not the result of bystander activation but represents an expansion of antigen-specific CD8 T cells. Peptide-MHC tetramer assays have shown promise in the study of the kinetics of primary and secondary immune responses and have resulted in better understanding of such concepts as immunodominance and clonal exhaustion.

An obviously attractive aspect of this technology is that tetramer staining can be combined with a variety of cell surface and intracellular phenotypic and functional markers. Indications that the phenotype of antigen-specific T cells varies among individuals and among different phases of the immune response are already present. In addition, tetramer-positive T cells can be sorted for further analysis, such as cytotoxicity assays or *in vitro* expansion. Tetramer-based technology has not only proven useful for the study of the immune response to infectious agents, it has also been applied to the study of oral tolerance, autoimmune conditions, and tumor immunology. It is likely that this highly sensitive and specific technology and other approaches that define the antigen-specific response will find many more applications and will lead to new discoveries and a reassessment of certain existing concepts.[58]

CONCLUSIONS

> ### On the Horizon
>
> - The combination of flow cytometry and mass spectrometry (cytof) expands the number of cell markers analyzed simultaneously ($\geq$35 currently performed), including extracellular and intracellular targets to provide an extensive evaluation of functional markers.
> - Flow cytometry utilizing spectral rather than conventional light analysis has the potential to allow more "colors" to be accurately evaluated without the need for complex compensation schemes to handle the overlapping light emissions from conventional fluorochromes. This could facilitate more extensive polychromatic studies to be performed easily in the clinical laboratory.

Flow cytometry has become readily available in clinical laboratories, and the application of this technology has moved forward along with significant improvements in instrumentation and the availability of an array of monoclonal reagents. Properly performed flow cytometry can provide rapid and accurate lymphocyte subpopulation identification. The primary clinical indications of immunophenotyping remain quantifying CD4 T-cell counts in HIV infection, lineage assignment in leukemias and lymphomas, evaluation of other hematological cell types, and assessment of CD34 expression to identify stem cells for transplantation. Additional uses include characterization of immune deficiency disorders, evaluation of immune-mediated inflammatory diseases, and assessment of patients after organ transplantation. Generally, immunophenotyping does not represent a diagnostic procedure but, rather, plays a part in the evaluation and understanding of complex disorders and the longitudinal evaluation of immunomodulatory therapy.

It is critical to recognize that immunophenotyping is a means of identifying cells but is not directed at cell function. The expansion of flow-cytometric techniques to evaluate intracellular characteristics, assess intracellular changes associated with activation, characterize apoptosis, and identify antigen-specific T cells has moved this technology into the cell function arena. These newer approaches expand the utility of flow cytometry as a valuable method for the characterization of various aspects of immune function.

This work was supported in part by the Intramural Research Program of the National Institutes of Health Clinical Center.

REFERENCES

1. Shapiro HM. *How Flow Cytometers Work.* 4th ed. Hoboken, NJ: Wiley; 2003.
2. Kachel V. *Hydrodynamic Properties of Flow Cytometry Instruments.* New York: Wiley Liss; 1990.
3. Thompson JM, Gralow JR, Levy R, et al. The optimal application of forward and ninety-degree light scatter in flow cytometry for the gating of mononuclear cells. *Cytometry.* 1985;6:401−406.
4. Goddard G, Martin JC, Graves SW, et al. Ultrasonic particle-concentration for sheathless focusing of particles for analysis in a flow cytometer. *Cytometry A.* 2006;69:66−74.
5. Ward M, Turner P, DeJohn M, et al. Fundamentals of acoustic cytometry. *Curr Protoc Cytom.* 2009;49:1.22.21−21.22.12.
6. Chattopadhyay PK, Hogerkorp CM, Roederer M. A chromatic explosion: the development and future of multiparameter flow cytometry. *Immunology.* 2008;125:441−449.
7. Perfetto SP, Chattopadhyay PK, Roederer M. Seventeen-colour flow cytometry: unravelling the immune system. *Nat Rev Immunol.* 2004;4:648−655.
8. Giepmans BN, Adams SR, Ellisman MH, et al. The fluorescent toolbox for assessing protein location and function. *Science.* 2006;312:217−224.
9. Chattopadhyay PK, Yu J, Roederer M. Application of quantum dots to multicolor flow cytometry. *Methods Mol Biol.* 2007;374:175−184.
10. Rabinovitch PS, June CH, Kavanagh TJ. Introduction to functional cell assays. *Ann N Y Acad Sci.* 1993;677:252−264.
11. Vowells SJ, Sekhsaria S, Malech HL, et al. Flow cytometric analysis of the granulocyte respiratory burst: a comparison study of fluorescent probes. *J Immunol Methods.* 1995;178:89−97.
12. Darzynkiewicz Z, Halicka HD, Zhao H. Analysis of cellular DNA content by flow and laser scanning cytometry. *Adv Exp Med Biol.* 2010;676:137−147.
13. Loken MR, Brosnan JM, Bach BA, et al. Establishing optimal lymphocyte gates for immunophenotyping by flow cytometry. *Cytometry.* 1990;11:453−459.
14. US Clinical and Laboratory Standards Institute. *Clinical Applications of Flow Cytometry: Quality Assurance and Immunophenotyping of Peripheral Blood Lymphocytes.* Villanova, PA: NCCLS Publication H24-T; 1992.
15. Stewart CC, Stewart SJ. Multiparameter data acquisition and analysis of leukocytes. *Methods Mol Biol.* 2004;263:45−66.
16. Parks DR, Roederer M, Moore WA. A new "Logicle" display method avoids deceptive effects of logarithmic scaling for low signals and compensated data. *Cytometry A.* 2006;69:541−551.
17. Roederer M, Moody MA. Polychromatic plots: graphical display of multidimensional data. *Cytometry A.* 2008;73:868−874.
18. Roederer M. Spectral compensation for flow cytometry: visualization artifacts, limitations, and caveats. *Cytometry.* 2001;45:194−205.
19. Owens MA, Vall HG, Hurley AA, et al. Validation and quality control of immunophenotyping in clinical flow cytometry. *J Immunol Methods.* 2000;243:33−50.
20. Schwartz A, Marti GE, Poon R, et al. Standardizing flow cytometry: a classification system of fluorescence standards used for flow cytometry. *Cytometry.* 1998;33:106−114.
21. Yamada M, Tamura N, Shirai T, et al. Flow cytometric analysis of lymphocyte subsets in the bronchoalveolar lavage fluid and peripheral blood of healthy volunteers. *Scand J Immunol.* 1986;24:559−565.
22. Reichert T, DeBruyere M, Deneys V, et al. Lymphocyte subset reference ranges in adult Caucasians. *Clin Immunol Immunopathol.* 1991;60:190−208.
23. Shearer WT, Rosenblatt HM, Gelman RS, et al. Lymphocyte subsets in healthy children from birth through 18 years of age: the pediatric AIDS clinical trials group P1009 study. *J Allergy Clin Immunol.* 2003;112:973−980.
24. Levi FA, Canon C, Touitou Y, et al. Seasonal modulation of the circadian time structure of circulating T and natural killer lymphocyte subsets from healthy subjects. *J Clin Invest.* 1988;81:407−413.
25. Fleisher TA, Oliveira JB. Autoimmune lymphoproliferative syndrome. *Isr Med Assoc J.* 2005;7:758−761.
26. Yarchoan R, Venzon DJ, Pluda JM, et al. CD4 count and the risk for death in patients infected with HIV receiving antiretroviral therapy. *Ann Intern Med.* 1991;115:184−189.
27. Sekhsaria S, Fleisher TA, Vowells S, et al. Granulocyte colony-stimulating factor recruitment of CD34+ progenitors to peripheral blood: impaired mobilization in chronic granulomatous disease and adenosine deaminase—deficient severe combined immunodeficiency disease patients. *Blood.* 1996;88:1104−1112.
28. Oliveira JB, Notarangelo LD, Fleisher TA. Applications of flow cytometry for the study of primary immune deficiencies. *Curr Opin Allergy Clin Immunol.* 2008;8:499−509.
29. Richardson AM, Moyer AM, Hasadri L, et al. Diagnostic tools for inborn errors of human immunity (Primary immunodeficiencies and immunodysregulatory diseases). *Curr Allergy Asthma Rep*; 2018:18−19. https://doi.org/10.1007/S11882-018-00770-1.
30. Wehr C, Kivioja T, Schmitt C, et al. The EUROclass trial: defining subgroups in common variable immunodeficiency. *Blood.* 2008;111:77−85.
31. Rosel AL, Scheibenbogen C, Schliesser U, et al. Classification of common variable immunodeficiencies using flow cytometry and a memory B-cell functional assay. *J Allergy Clin Immunol.* 2014;135:198−208.

32. Bonilla FA, Barlan I, Chapel H, et al. International consensus document (ICON): common variable immunodeficiency disorders. *J Allergy Clin Immunol Pract.* 2016;4:38–59.

33. Etzioni A. Defects in the leukocyte adhesion cascade. *Clin Rev Allergy Immunol.* 2010;38:54–60.

34. Schuurhuis GJ, Heuser M, Freeman S, et al. Minimal/measurable residual disease in AML: a consensus document from the European leukemia net MRD working party. *Blood.* 2018;131:1275–1291.

35. Berliner N, Ault KA, Martin P, et al. Detection of clonal excess in lymphoproliferative disease by kappa/lambda analysis: correlation with immunoglobulin gene DNA rearrangement. *Blood.* 1986;67:80–85.

36. Pilch H, Hohn H, Freitag K, et al. Improved assessment of T-cell receptor (TCR) VB repertoire in clinical specimens: combination of TCR- CDR3 spectratyping with flow cytometry-based TCR VB frequency analysis. *Clin Diagn Lab Immunol.* 2002;9:257–266.

37. Sallusto F, Geginat J, Lanzavecchia A. Central memory and effector memory T cell subsets: function, generation, and maintenance. *Annu Rev Immunol.* 2004;22:745–763.

38. Avery DT, Ellyard JI, Mackay F, et al. Increased expression of CD27 on activated human memory B cells correlates with their commitment to the plasma cell lineage. *J Immunol.* 2005;174:4034–4042.

39. Alter G, Malenfant JM, Altfeld M. CD107a as a functional marker for the identification of natural killer activity. *J Immunol Methods.* 2004;294:15–22.

40. Marcenaro S, Gall F, Martini S, et al. Analysis of natural killer-cell function in familial hemophagocytic lymphohistiocytosis (FHL): defective CD107a surface expression heralds Munc13-4 defect and discriminates between genetic subtypes of the disease. *Blood.* 2006;108:2316–2323.

41. Mardiney 3rd M, Brown MR, Fleisher TA. Measurement of T-cell CD69 expression: a rapid and efficient means to assess mitogen- or antigen-induced proliferative capacity in normals. *Cytometry.* 1996;26:305–310.

42. Allsopp CE, Langhorne J. Assessing antigen-specific proliferation and cytokine responses using flow cytometry. *Methods Mol Med.* 2002;72:409–421.

43. Slezak SE, Horan PK. Cell-mediated cytotoxicity. A highly sensitive and informative flow cytometric assay. *J Immunol Methods.* 1989;117:205–214.

44. Yu Y, Arora A, Min W, et al. EdU incorporation is an alternative non-radioactive assay to [(3)H]thymidine uptake for in vitro measurement of mice T-cell proliferations. *J Immunol Methods.* 2009;350:29–35.

45. Fleisher TA, Dorman SE, Anderson JA, et al. Detection of intracellular phosphorylated STAT-1 by flow cytometry. *Clin Immunol.* 1999;90:425–430.

46. Vowells SJ, Fleisher TA, Sekhsaria S, et al. Genotype-dependent variability in flow cytometric evaluation of reduced nicotinamide adenine dinucleotide phosphate oxidase function in patients with chronic granulomatous disease. *J Pediatr.* 1996;128:104–107.

47. Heim KF, Fleisher TA, Stroncek DF, et al. The relationship between alloimmunization and posttransfusion granulocyte survival: experience in a chronic granulomatous disease cohort. *Transfusion.* 2001;51:1154–1162.

48. Kuhns DB, Alvord WG, Heller T, et al. Residual NADPH oxidase and survival in chronic granulomatous disease. *N Engl J Med.* 2010;363:2600–2610.

49. Foster B, Prussin C, Liu F, et al. Detection of intracellular cytokines by flow cytometry. *Curr Protoc Immunol.* 2007; Chapter 6:Unit 6.24.

50. Suni MA, Picker LJ, Maino VC. Detection of antigen-specific T cell cytokine expression in whole blood by flow cytometry. *J Immunol Methods.* 1998;212:89–98.

51. Shankey TV, Rabinovitch PS, Bagwell B, et al. Guidelines for implementation of clinical DNA cytometry. International Society for Analytical Cytology. *Cytometry.* 1993; 14:472–477.

52. Braylan RC, Benson NA, Nourse V, et al. Correlated analysis of cellular DNA, membrane antigens and light scatter of human lymphoid cells. *Cytometry.* 1982;2: 337–343.

53. Rothaeusler K, Baumgarth N. Assessment of cell proliferation by 5-bromodeoxyuridine (BrdU) labeling for multicolor flow cytometry. *Curr Protoc Cytom.* 2007; Chapter 7: Unit 7.31.

54. Gong J, Bhatia U, Traganos F, et al. Expression of cyclins A, D2 and D3 in individual normal mitogen stimulated lymphocytes and in MOLT-4 leukemic cells analyzed by multiparameter flow cytometry. *Leukemia.* 1995;9: 893–899.

55. Telford WG, Komoriya A, Packard BZ, et al. Multiparametric analysis of apoptosis by flow cytometry. *Methods Mol Biol.* 2011;699:203–227.

56. Altman JD, Moss PA, Goulder PJ, et al. Phenotypic analysis of antigen-specific T lymphocytes. *Science.* 1996;274: 94–96.

57. Mallone R, Nepom GT. MHC Class II tetramers and the pursuit of antigen-specific T cells: define, deviate, delete. *Clin Immunol.* 2004;110:232–242.

58. Kern F, LiPira G, Gratama JW, et al. Measuring Ag-specific immune responses: understanding immunopathogenesis and improving diagnostics in infectious disease, autoimmunity and cancer. *Trends Immunol.* 2005;26:477–484.

CHAPTER 3

Evaluation of Lymphocyte Function

ROSHINI SARAH ABRAHAM

The immune response is mediated by a complex network of cells, soluble and membrane-bound biological mediators and receptors interacting within the context of specific tissues and organs to protect against pathogens. Although the immune system has been broadly divided into innate and adaptive components, there is considerable overlap and interaction between the two, despite the highly specialized functions and kinetics of each in the immune response. T and B cells form the pillar of the adaptive immune response, whereas natural killer (NK) cells are the effector lymphocytes of the innate immune response. There are approximately 2×10^{12} lymphocytes in the body, and typically the response to a foreign antigen is in the context of initial activation of innate immune components. T cells recognize antigen primarily in the context of antigen-specific T-cell receptors (TCRs) and specific peptides presented by molecules of the major histocompatibility complex (MHC), either class I or class II. T cells are also capable of responding nonspecifically to polyclonal stimulators, such as mitogens (*in vitro*) or superantigens (*in vivo*) that do not initiate an antigen-specific proliferative response. T cells upon activation also produce cytokines that are crucial to their effector functions including activating B cells and inducing antibody production, promoting differentiation of cytotoxic T cells, activating macrophages, and promoting activation and migration of inflammatory cells. Cytokines play a role in the induction of the T-cell response when produced by antigen-presenting cells (APCs) at the time of antigen recognition. B cells recognize antigen directly via the B-cell receptor (involving surface immunoglobulin) and produce antibodies with help from T cells (T-dependent antigens) or from the innate immune system (T-independent antigens). More recently, the granularity of the antibody response has been further delineated, and T-dependent antibody responses are divided into type 1, with help provided by T-follicular helper cells (Tfhs), and type 2, with help provided by NKTfh cells. Similarly, T-independent responses are classified into three groups: type 1, induced by recognition of microbial antigens by the toll-like receptors (TLRs) in the absence of Bruton's tyrosine kinase (BTK); type 2, which requires the presence of BTK; and type 3, which has neutrophil B-helper cells.[1,2]

Regulatory (Treg) cells play a critical role in the control of both physiological and pathological immune responses in a variety of contexts. Treg cells exert a direct inhibitory effect on the development of autoimmune disease because their absence leads to the development of a severe phenotype, as manifested by the FOXP3 deficiency, IPEX (immune dysfunction/polyendocrinopathy/enteropathy/X-linked).[3] Treg cells can suppress the proliferation of antigen-stimulated naïve T cells, as demonstrated by *in vitro* studies, and induction of FOXP3 in conventional naïve T cells imparts suppressive function *in vitro* and *in vivo*, resulting in the generation of induced regulatory T (iTreg) cells.[4] Besides producing antibodies to neutralize pathogens and presenting antigen to T cells, B cells also exert immunomodulatory control of the immune response, primarily via interleukin (IL)-10 production. IL-10-producing B cells, classified as regulatory B (Breg) cells, play an important role in immune homeostasis and in protection against autoimmune responses and inflammatory damage. Breg cells, in addition to producing IL-10, secrete other cytokines that act on other effector T-cell subsets, Tregs, APCs such as dendritic cells (DCs), and macrophages.

NK cells are considered to be innate immune effector cells, but they straddle the threshold of innate and

Core Laboratory Technologies in Clinical Immunology. https://doi.org/10.1016/B978-0-323-66149-2.00003-7

adaptive immunity. NK cells are directly involved in cytotoxicity and cytokine secretion upon activation, but they also function indirectly by regulating APC and the effector T cells' response. NK cell activation is controlled by synergistic signals from activating and inhibitory receptors.[5] The characteristics, responses, and assays to measure the activity and function of each of these subsets are described in detail in the following sections.

T-CELL RESPONSE

T cells form the cellular arm of the adaptive immune response, and each T cell has unique specificity derived from the presence of a functional, antigen-recognizing receptor on the cell surface. Naïve T cells derived from the thymus can migrate through the peripheral circulation and secondary lymphoid tissues (spleen and lymph nodes), but they cannot effectively participate in the immune response to pathogens. To do so, naïve T cells must undergo a defined process of cellular activation, which involves recognition of antigen by the TCR in the context of MHC molecules. The majority of circulating T cells express the α/β TCR, whereas a smaller proportion of cells express the γ/δ TCR. On the surface of the T cell, the TCR associates with the CD3 complex, comprised of four distinct subunits (γ, δ, ϵ, and ζ); the cytosolic components of the CD3 complex are involved in the intracellular propagation of signals after ligation of the TCR. Besides the CD3 complex, the TCR also clusters with a CD4 or CD8 coreceptor, depending on the type of T cell; CD4 T cells recognize antigen (Ag) in the context of MHC class II, whereas CD8 T cells recognize antigen presented on MHC class I. The first signal or "cognate" signal, which is recognition of peptide-MHC complex by the TCR, results in actin-mediated reorganization of the cytoskeleton in both the T cell and APC to form the immunological synapse (Fig. 3.1). The synapse consists of the TCR along with other costimulatory molecules and adhesion receptors, which results in the formation of a large macromolecular structure called the supramolecular activation complex (SMAC). The unique organization of the SMAC results in prolonged and stronger intracellular interactions and appropriate downstream signaling activity, including phosphorylation of the CD3 receptor components. The complete culmination of the TCR-induced signals results in IL-2 production and secretion, which drives T-cell proliferation in an autocrine and paracrine manner.

It is important to recognize that various T-cell processes and stages of differentiation are specifically regulated by metabolic pathways.[6] For example, naïve T cells rely on oxidative phosphorylation for their metabolism, with additional glycolytic metabolism during times of proliferation. On the other hand, activated effector T cells demonstrate aerobic glycolysis and increased oxidative phosphorylation. T-helper cell-1 (Th1), Th2, and Th17 CD4 effector T cells use glycolytic metabolism, whereas regulatory T-cell and memory T-cell development is enhanced by fatty acid oxidation and catabolic metabolism. In particular, memory T cells are quiescent and mainly use oxidative phosphorylation; however, on antigenic rechallenge, the use of oxidative phosphorylation and glycolysis is rapidly facilitated.[6] While naïve T-cell activation and differentiation into effector cells are essential for a normal immune response during exposure to acute an antigenic challenge, chronic antigenic stimulation via persistent antigen exposure and/or inflammation causes an alteration of memory T-cell differentiation, resulting in a state of T-cell exhaustion. During T-cell exhaustion there is a progressive diminution of effector functions, along with upregulation of several inhibitory receptors, metabolic changes, and a failure to transition to a quiescent state and to obtain an antigen-independent memory T-cell homeostatic response. Exhausted T cells have only a limited ability to clear pathogens or tumors; however, there is some evidence that this is a reversible phenomenon, at least at a global level.[7]

Clinical Relevance
Lymphocyte Function Evaluation

- Assessment of lymphocyte function typically refers to measurement of T-cell function via cellular proliferation to nonspecific and specific stimuli; however, it is much broader and more comprehensive and refers to any method that assesses any of the various effector or regulatory aspects of any lymphocyte subset.
- The robustness of clinical interpretation of lymphocyte function assays is dependent on the analytical procedure, sample type, timing of collection, and clinical context, among other factors. Assays performed in clinical diagnostic immunology laboratories are standardized to minimize inconsistencies in these variables.

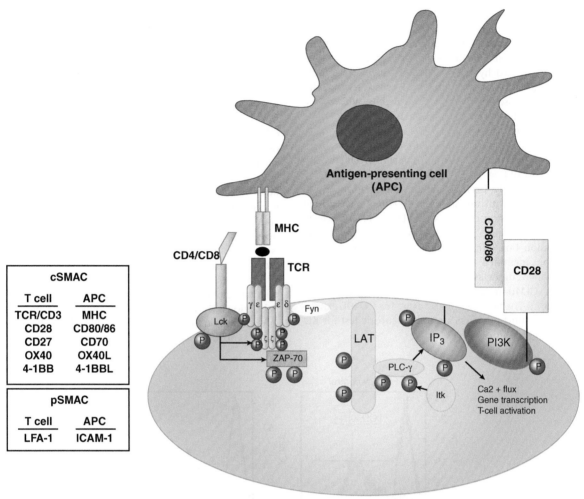

FIG. 3.1 Mechanism of T-Cell Activation. T cells recognize antigen in the context of major histocompatibility complex (MHC) molecules on antigen-presenting cells (APCs). Sustained interaction between a T cell and APC results in the formation of the immunological synapse with membrane reorganization and ordering of key molecules on both cells into a supramolecular activation complex (SMAC) comprised of c (central) SMAC and p (peripheral) SMAC. Cognate interaction with appropriate costimulatory signals results in intracellular signaling events that ultimately result in T-cell activation. *LAT*, linker for activation of T cells; *PLC-*γ, phospholipase C-gamma; *TCR*, T-cell receptor; *IP3*, inositol 1, 4, 5 triphosphate; *P*, phosphorylation; *PI3K*, phosphatidylinositol 3′-hydroxyl kinase; *Lck* and *Fyn*, Src-family nonreceptor protein tyrosine kinases; *Itk*, IL-2-inducible T-cell kinase; *ZAP-70*, ζ-chain-associated protein kinase 70. (Adapted from Figure 1, Pennock ND, et al. *Adv Physiol Educ* 2013;37:273–83.)

ASSESSMENT OF T-CELL FUNCTION VIA ACTIVATION MARKERS

Activation of T cells results in the expression of several induced markers, which can be used to ascertain the competence of T cells participating in the immune response. These include CD69, CD154 (CD40L), MHC class II, and CD25, which are expressed in a sequential manner and can be assessed by flow cytometry (Chapter 2).[8] In contrast to *in vivo* activation of T cells and subsequent expression of these markers, *in vitro* assessment of T-cell function involves activation of T cells with nonspecific and polyclonal stimulants such as phorbol myristate acetate (PMA) or phytohemagglutinin (PHA), which results in expression of these markers in a kinetically regulated fashion.[8] The expression of CD40L on activated T cells, besides being useful as a global marker for T-cell activation, is used more specifically for the diagnosis of a primary immunodeficiency, X-linked hyper-IgM syndrome or CD40L deficiency. CD40L on activated CD4 T cells interacts with CD40, expressed constitutively on B cells, and participates in isotype (class)-switching as well as providing costimulatory help to T cells. The expression of CD40L on activated CD4 T cells can easily be ascertained in the laboratory using an *in vitro* T-cell stimulation protocol (Fig. 3.2). In this assay, CD69 is used as a control for early T-cell activation. The majority of patients (80%) with mutations in *CD40LG* have absent protein expression on activated CD4 T cells; however, 20% of mutations may remain permissive for protein expression but with aberrant function. These patients can be identified by incorporating an additional component in the assay using a soluble form of the receptor CD40-muIg to assess binding of the ligand (Fig. 3.2). The flow cytometric assay for CD40L expression and function offers a rapid diagnostic test for XL-Hyper IgM syndrome.[9]

DETERMINATION OF CELLULAR VIABILITY IN LYMPHOCYTES

The flow cytometry–based assays also allow determination of viable cells in the sample after peripheral blood mononuclear cell (PBMC) isolation from whole heparinized blood, which is particularly important in the interpretation of results (Fig. 3.3). The use of annexin V in a flow cytometry assay enables visualization of apoptotic cells. An early event in cell apoptosis is the translocation of membrane phosphatidylserine (PS) to the cell surface. Annexin V is a calcium (Ca^{2+})-dependent phospholipid-binding protein, which has a strong affinity for PS, and a fluorochrome-conjugated reagent directed at annexin V is used in a flow assay. In addition to visualizing apoptotic cells, dead cells can be assessed by simultaneously using 7-amino-actinomycin-D (7-AAD), which is a membrane-impermeable dye that is generally excluded from viable cells. When internalized into dying or dead cells, it binds to double-stranded DNA by intercalating between base pairs in guanine (G)-cytosine (C)-rich regions. These two dyes can be combined to provide information on the proportion of viable cells in the starting cell mixture for proliferation assays (Fig. 3.3).

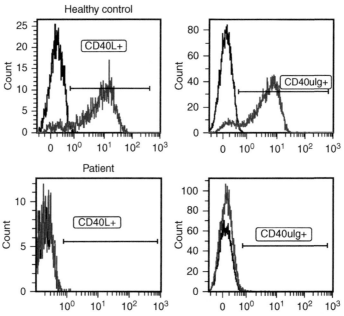

FIG. 3.2 CD40L Expression on Activated CD4 T Cells. CD40L is an early activation marker expressed on CD4 T cells, and it is important for T-cell costimulation and isotype class-switching. In healthy individuals, on T-cell activation, CD40L (CD154) is expressed on the cell surface of CD4 T cells and is capable of binding a soluble form of the receptor CD40µIg, which enables assessment of its function *in vitro* (top panel). In patients with X-linked hyper-IgM syndrome due to CD40L deficiency, either there is no protein expression of CD40L on the cell surface and therefore no binding to the soluble receptor (lower panel) or, as is the case with 20% of patients, the CD40L expressed on the cell surface is nonfunctional and cannot bind to the receptor (CD40µIg).

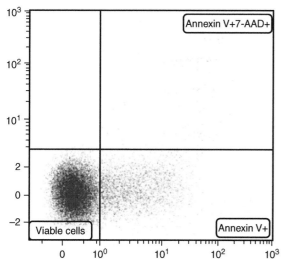

FIG. 3.3 Determination of Cellular Viability for Lymphocyte Function Studies. For all functional assessments of immune response, it is essential and useful to measure the proportion of viable cells at the initiation of the analysis and even at the end of the analysis, if required. Measurement of cell apoptosis and death can be achieved by flow cytometry analysis of annexin V positivity (apoptotic) and annexin V 7-amino-actinomycin-D (7-AAD) dual positive (dead) cells. Cells that are negative for both these markers are viable cells, and their frequency can be assessed in the flow assay.

ASSESSMENT OF T-CELL COMPETENCE VIA PROLIFERATION

Mitogens are very potent stimulators of T-cell activation and induce polyclonal T-cell proliferation. It has been suggested that mitogens can induce T-cell proliferative responses even if the lymphocytes are incapable of responding adequately to antigenic (physiological) stimuli. Therefore abnormal T-cell responses to mitogens are considered a diagnostically less sensitive but more specific test of aberrant T-cell function. Lectin mitogens bind to the TCR, thereby activating quiescent T cells. Mitogenic stimulation induces increased intracellular calcium (Ca^{2+}) in T cells, which is essential for T-cell proliferation. Whereas PHA is a strong T-cell mitogen (Fig. 3.4), PWM is a weak T-cell mitogen that also induces B-cell activation and proliferation with a different time line for maximal stimulation. Mitogens such as PHA activate T cells by binding to cell membrane glycoproteins, including the TCR-CD3 complex.

In addition, there are a number of mitogenic or comitogenic antibodies, including those directed against the CD3 coreceptor that can stimulate T-cell proliferation. Typically, anti-CD3 antibodies provide an initial activation signal and provide a variable proliferative response (Fig. 3.5). Addition of a costimulatory antibody (anti-CD28) to anti-CD3 results in enhanced proliferation (Fig. 3.5). An exogenous T-cell growth factor, such as IL-2, can also be used as an alternate to anti-CD28 costimulation, and in patients with suspected IL-2 receptor (IL-2R)-associated signaling defects, it may be more helpful from a diagnostic perspective than the use of anti-CD28 (Fig. 3.5). IL-2, an autocrine cytokine, has been demonstrated to be critical in T-cell proliferation and in regulation of T-cell growth through binding to a heterotrimeric receptor complex consisting of 3 chains—α, β, and γ (IL-2Rα, IL-2Rβ, and IL-2Rγ)—on the surface of T cells. Triggering of the TCR leads to synthesis of IL-2 in certain T-cell subsets with induction of high-affinity IL-2Rs on antigen- or mitogen-activated T cells; the binding of IL-2 to the IL-2R ultimately leads to T-cell proliferation. The use of exogenous IL-2 in association with anti-CD3 allows discrimination of T cells that cannot proliferate to other mitogenic signals but can respond to a potent growth factor such as IL-2.

Antigens including candida antigen (CA) and tetanus toxoid (TT) have been widely used to measure antigen-specific recall (anamnestic) T-cell responses when assessing cellular immunity. In fact, this may be more revealing about cellular immune compromise than assessing the response of lymphocytes to mitogens because the latter can induce T-cell proliferative responses even if those T cells are incapable of responding adequately to antigenic (physiological) stimuli. Therefore abnormal T-cell responses to antigens are considered a diagnostically more sensitive, but less specific, test of aberrant T-cell function. Antigens used in recall assays measure the ability of T cells bearing specific TCRs to respond to antigenic peptides presented by APCs. The antigens used for assessment of the cellular immune response are selected to represent antigens, seen by a majority of the population either through natural exposure (CA) or as a result of vaccination (TT) (Fig. 3.6).

In addition to measuring cellular proliferation as a readout for T-cell function, the production of cytokines by activated T cells is another important component for evaluating T-cell functional activity. T cells typically are

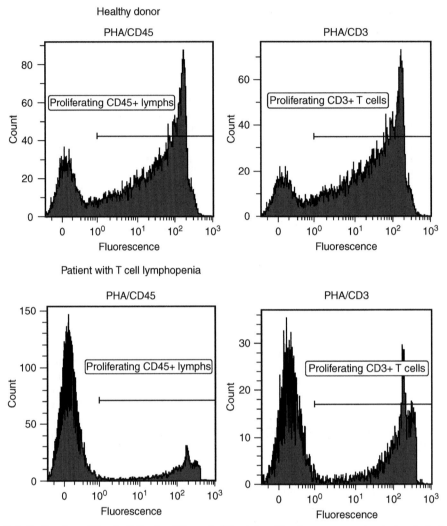

FIG. 3.4 Proliferation of T cells Following Mitogenic Stimulation. T cells can respond polyclonally to *in vitro* stimulation with various mitogens. T-cell proliferation assessment by flow cytometry allows analysis in total lymphocytes (CD45$^+$) and T cells (CD3$^+$). The top panel demonstrates T-cell proliferation to phytohemagglutinin (PHA) in both cell subsets. In patients with T-cell lymphopenia, where cellular dilution may be a concern, single-cell analysis by flow cytometry allows discrimination of functional versus nonfunctional T cells. In the lower panel, a patient with T-cell lymphopenia has abnormal proliferation when total lymphocytes are assessed; however, the response is normal when the T-cell compartment is specifically evaluated. Therefore this patient, who would have been classified as abnormal based only on the CD45$^+$ lymphocyte response, can be reclassified as having normal T-cell proliferation based on the CD3$^+$ T-cell response, but with significant T-cell lymphopenia.

not monofunctional, producing a single cytokine on activation; rather, they are multi- or polyfunctional, and the range of cytokines are produced in a sequential manner rather than simultaneously, although a population of stimulated T cells will have individual T cells producing different cytokines in a temporally regulated manner. These cytokines can be measured by intracellular flow cytometry after T-cell activation

with mitogens, in both CD4 and CD8 T-cell subsets or alternatively in the culture supernatant of activated cells. Typically, the cytokines measured in *in vitro* stimulation assays include IL-2, interferon (IFN)-γ, IL-4, IL-5, IL-6, IL-17, and tumor necrosis factor (TNF)-α.

The process of T-cell activation as described above results in IL-2 production that drives T-cell

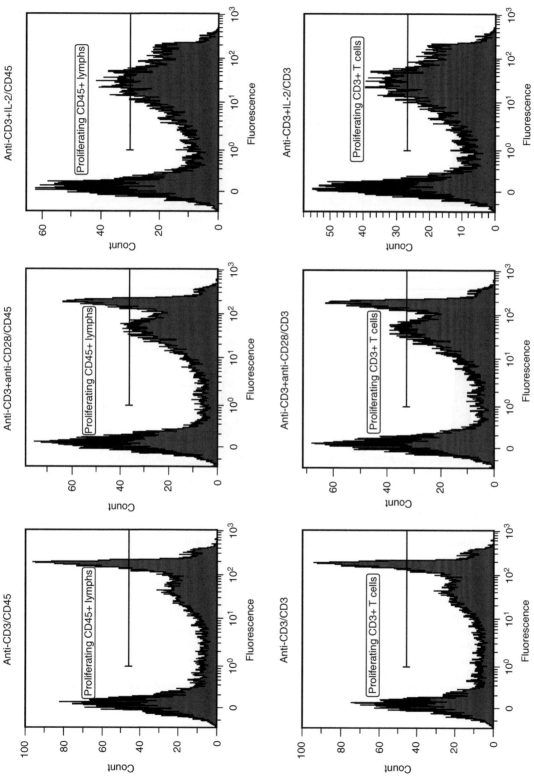

FIG. 3.5 Proliferation of T Cells Secondary to Anti-CD3 Stimulants. Assessment of T-cell proliferation to CD3 coreceptor cross-linking provides a more physiological, yet global, evaluation of T-cell function. T cells are stimulated with either soluble anti-CD3 alone or soluble anti-CD3 plus anti-CD28 or with soluble anti-CD3 plus interleukin (IL)-2. In each case, proliferation is measured in total CD45+ lymphocytes and CD3+ T cells. An example of anti-CD3-stimulated T-cell response is shown in a healthy donor.

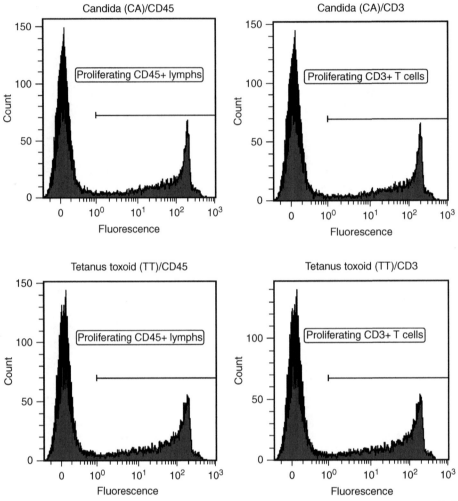

FIG. 3.6 Determination of Antigen-Induced T-Cell Proliferation. Antigens such as candida antigen (CA) and tetanus toxoid (TT) are frequently used to assess antigen-specific T-cell function. As with mitogens and anti-CD3 stimulation, proliferation is measured in total CD45$^+$ lymphocytes and CD3$^+$ T cells. An example in a healthy donor is shown.

proliferation. Measuring T-cell proliferation after stimulation *in vitro* with various specific and nonspecific stimuli has been a staple of the diagnostic immunology repertoire for several decades. T-cell proliferation assays can be divided into three categories: use of nonspecific mitogenic stimuli such as PHA, pokeweed mitogen (PWM), and concanavalin A (Con A); physiological global stimuli based on CD3 coreceptor cross-linking (using anti-CD3, either soluble or bead-bound) with or without CD28 cross-linking (using anti-CD28, either soluble or bead-bound); and with or without exogenous IL-2. Antigen-specific stimulation depends on the use of common recall antigens.

Key Concepts
T-Cell Activation and Function

- Cognate recognition of peptide major histocompatibility complex (MHC) on the APC by the T-cell receptor results in formation of the immunological synapse.
- Activated T cells express early activation markers, such as CD69 and CD40L. Other T-cell activation markers include CD25 and MHC class II (human leukocyte antigen–D related [HLA-DR]).
- T cells can be stimulated to proliferate using nonspecific stimulants such as plant lectins (mitogens) and cross-linking of the CD3 coreceptor, along

The commonly used method for assessing T-cell proliferation for decades involved measurement of ^{3}H-thymidine (^{3}H-T) incorporated into the DNA of proliferating cells. The results are expressed as either counts per minute (cpm) or disintegrations per minute (dpm) of both activated and nonactivated cells (background) cultured for a fixed period of time, usually 72 hours for mitogens. A reference range based on proliferation results from a group of control subjects should be provided along with the patients' results (both background and poststimulation results). Although this method remains widely employed, several disadvantages exist, including but not limited to the use of radioactive material (^{3}H-T); its inability to discriminate responder cell subsets or to account for cellular dilution, which is particularly relevant in the context of T-cell lymphopenia; and the lack of information on the contribution of cell death after stimulation and its impact on the final result. To overcome the intrinsic shortcomings of the ^{3}H-T method, newer flow cytometry assays are currently being used in the clinical diagnostic setting and are gaining popularity because of the additional information they provide.

The flow cytometric methods for measuring cell proliferation include the use of fluorescent dyes to identify proliferating cells. One of the more commonly used dyes, carboxyfluorescein diacetate succinimidyl ester (CFSE), must be carefully used when measuring lymphocyte proliferation *in vitro* since it can be toxic to cells and nonoptimal labeling conditions can impact measurement of cell proliferation and interpretation of results. CFSE is a fluorescent cell membrane—permeable dye similar in physical properties to the commonly used fluorochrome, fluorescein isothiocyanate (FITC). During cell proliferation, the intensity of staining in daughter cells is half that of parent cells, allowing visualization of the number of rounds of cell divisions associated with the successive decrease in fluorescence. The disadvantages to using CFSE in the clinical laboratory are its

photo-instability, limitation in the number of cell divisions being identified ($\leq$7 cell divisions), and interpretation requires measuring loss of signal rather than gain of signal. In addition, as noted above, CFSE at concentrations of 37 nM to 10 μM can be toxic to cells resulting in increased cell death. Furthermore, it can modulate expression of activation markers, resulting in a decrease in CD69, HLA-DR, and CD25 expression. Finally, it has been reported that there is an increase in the number of false-positive results with CFSE making it suboptimal for measuring lymphocyte proliferation in patients with severe cellular immunodeficiencies. Alternatives to CFSE include related compounds, such as Cell Trace Violet (CTV) and Cell Proliferation Dye eFluor 670 (CPD), which have different excitation and emission spectra compared with CFSE. These dyes also can be used for tracking lymphocyte proliferation status *in vivo*, in animal models, permitting measurement of up to 11 cell divisions.*

Another alternative to tritiated thymidine is the use of a thymidine analog, 5-ethynyl-2'-deoxyuridine (Edu®), which can combine with a fluorescent azide in a copper-catalyzed cycloaddition reaction (referred to as "Click" chemistry) and permits flow cytometric evaluation of lymphocyte proliferative responses by assessing its incorporation into cellular DNA. Edu® labeling has been shown to be a fast and sensitive method for measuring cell proliferation and also facilitates identification of dividing cells. It is relatively more photostable than CFSE and is added to cells after completion of the stimulation period with the measurement being comparable to the thymidine method in regards to a gain of signal in the endpoint. The Edu® assay has not shown the limitations of the CFSE method in the clinical laboratory and has been used to evaluate lymphocyte proliferation in a spectrum of patients, including those with severe combined immunodeficiencies (SCIDs). In fact, this assay has been particularly useful in discriminating between functional T cells and nonfunctional T cells in the context of severe T cell lymphopenia, which cannot be achieved with the standard thymidine assay (Figs. 3.4—3.6). All the proliferation data shown in this chapter utilize this Edu®-based measurement of T cell proliferation, and results are typically provided for both CD45 bright positive (total lymphocytes) and CD3 T cells, with the former being more representative of the data generated with the standard thymidine assay.*

---

*This section has been reproduced in part with permission from ASM Press (Abraham RS, Lymphocyte Activation) (copyright permission obtained).

DETERMINATION OF CELL-MEDIATED CYTOTOXICITY

CD8 T cells are considered the representative cytotoxic T cell in the immune system, and cellular cytotoxicity is a mechanism to eliminate cells infected with intracellular pathogens, allogeneic cells, or tumor cells. CD8 T cells, like CD4 T cells, recognize antigen via the TCR and kill target cells via cytotoxic protein granule exocytosis and/or cytokine production. Over the past few decades, the cytotoxic potential of CD4 T cells has been described, particularly in viral infections. Although cytotoxic CD4 T cells are rare in the circulation of healthy individuals (<2%), they can account for substantial proportions of total CD4 T cells in certain viral infections, including but not limited to HIV.[10] The CD4 cytotoxic T cells appear to be a lineage of memory CD4 T cells that contain cytotoxic granules with perforin and granzymes, and they are thought to arise in the context of chronic or potent activation with viral infections such as cytomegalovirus (CMV), Epstein-Barr virus (EBV), human immunodeficiency virus (HIV), or certain autoimmune diseases.[11]

Key Concepts
Cellular Cytotoxicity

- CD8$^+$ T cells and natural killer (NK) cells are involved in killing of cellular targets and contain intracellular granules with cytotoxic proteins, such as perforin and granzymes.
- Cytotoxic CD4$^+$ T cells are a subset of memory T cells with cytolytic potential and are usually observed in circulation in the context of chronic viral infections, *e.g.*, cytomegalovirus (CMV), human immunodeficiency virus (HIV).
- Tetramer-based assays have been used to quantify and delineate function of antigen-specific CD8$^+$ T cells (also CD4$^+$ T cells).
- Cellular degranulation results in expression of CD107a on the cell surface of CD8$^+$ T cells and NK cells and is often used as a surrogate of cytotoxic activity.
- NK cells recognize target cells that lack major histocompatibility complex (MHC) class I, *e.g.*, viral cells or tumor cells that have downregulated MHC class I.
- The majority of circulating NK cells are cytotoxic (CD3$^-$CD16^{++}CD56$^{+/-}$), while a minority are cytokine producing (CD3$^-$CD56^{++}).
- Interleukin (IL)-2 augments NK cell–mediated cytotoxicity (lymphokine-activated killing) and also induces interferon (IFN)-γ secretion by NK cells.
- Regulatory T cells control NK cell activation and cytotoxic function by limiting availability of IL-2.

Cellular cytotoxic activity has been conventionally measured by release of chromium (^{51}Cr) from labeled target (T) cells cultured with various ratios of effector (E) cells (varied E:T ratio). The percentage lysis is developed using the level of radioactivity in the supernatant of target cells in comparison to controls consisting of target cells cultured alone (no lysis) and target cells exposed to hypotonic conditions (*e.g.*, distilled water, saponin) representing 100% lysis. Similar to the radioactive assay for measuring T-cell proliferation described previously, there are several limitations to the radioactive cytotoxicity assay, including the hazard of radioactive material, the difficulty in labeling target cells with ^{51}Cr, and bulk quantitation of cytotoxic activity, which does not allow single cell–specific analysis. Alternative assays have been developed, including flow cytometry and ELISPOT-based methods.[12] More recently, a method of assessing human CD8 T-cell cytotoxicity has been described in which both the effector and target cells are primary cells (in contrast to using cell lines as target cells).[13] In this particular assay, autologous B cells isolated from PBMC are used as target cells and cocultured with antigen-specific CD8 effector cells. The killing of the fluorescently labeled target B cells (see section on NK Cell Cytotoxicity) is used to estimate cytotoxic activity. Antigen-specific effector cells are quantified in the total CD8 T-cell pool using MHC-peptide tetramers.[13]

A tetramer-based approach to quantifying and measuring function of CMV-specific CD8 T cells has been available in the clinical diagnostic immunology laboratory for over a decade (Fig. 3.7). However, the limitation of the tetramer approach in the clinical diagnostic setting is that it is constrained by the number of HLA-peptide tetramer (multimer) combinations that are available for use with a particular antigen (*e.g.*, CMV, EBV). It also requires *a priori* knowledge of the patient's HLA genotype, and very often it does not incorporate a comprehensive assessment of the CD8 and CD4 cytotoxic T-cell response. Although some laboratories use only a quantitative approach to determine immune competence to pathogens, such as CMV with the tetramer assay, more comprehensive assays are available that also provide a functional assessment of these antigen-specific CD8 T cells (Fig. 3.7).

An alternative approach is to evaluate for cytotoxic function by assessing degranulation through evaluation of CD107a expression by the effector T cell (described in further detail in the section on NK cell function) and/or evaluating IFN-γ production by activated cytotoxic CD8 T cells. As a positive control, CD8 T cells are polyclonally stimulated with PMA and ionomycin,

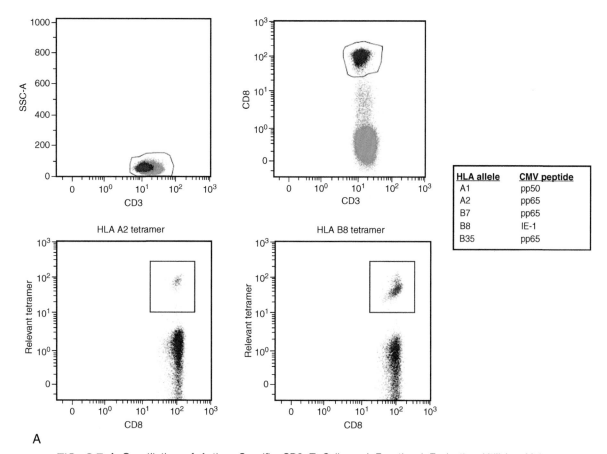

HLA allele	CMV peptide
A1	pp50
A2	pp65
B7	pp65
B8	IE-1
B35	pp65

A

FIG. 3.7 A Quantitation of Antigen-Specific CD8 T Cells and Functional Evaluation Utilizing Major Histocompatibility Complex (MHC) Class I Tetramers. The tetramer (multimer) technology has been useful for accurate quantitation of antigen-specific CD8 (or CD4 T cells, if MHC class II tetramers are used). The top panels show identification of CD3$^+$ T cells from total lymphocytes and subsequent segregation into CD3$^+$CD8$^+$ T cells. In this assay, cytomegalovirus (CMV)-specific CD8$^+$ T cells are quantitated using five MHC class I tetramers (human leukocyte antigen [HLA] A1, A2, B7, B8, and B35), each recognizing a unique CMV peptide from three major CMV antigenic proteins (pp50, pp65, and IE-1) as listed in the box. Based on the HLA class I haplotype of the individual, one or more tetramers are used for stimulation. The bottom panels show an example of a patient with HLA A2–specific CMV-CD8$^+$ T cells and another patient with HLA B8–specific CMV-CD8$^+$ T cells. These CMV-specific CD8$^+$ T cells can be assessed for functional capacity by gating on the tetramer-positive CD8$^+$ T cells and then measuring degranulation (CD107a expression) and inteferon (IFN)-γ production after *in vitro* stimulation with the specific CMV peptide (B). The data are shown for CD107a expression and IFN-γ production in unstimulated CMV-CD8$^+$ T cells and peptide-stimulated CMV-CD8$^+$ T cells.

and the same markers (CD107a expression and IFN-γ production) are measured. Approximately 10—60% of CD8 T cells in healthy adults are activated to express CD107a and to secrete IFN-γ under these conditions. An approach that avoids the use of tetramers involves the stimulation of patient-specific PBMC with overlapping peptide pools of the specific antigen and, subsequently, the evaluation of the CD8 and CD4 T cells

that proliferate in response to antigenic stimulation. These T cells can also be assessed for cytotoxic potential by measuring intracellular perforin and granzyme expression as well as degranulation (CD107a expression) after stimulation.[8]

A CMV-specific assay has been developed that measures IFN-γ production in response to CD8 T-cell stimulation with a pool of MHC class I—restricted

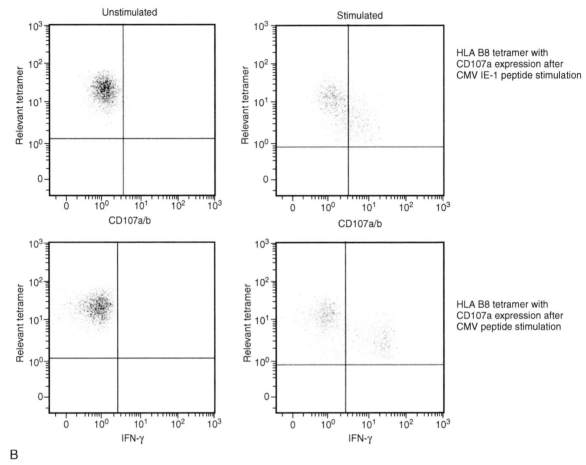

FIG. 3.7 **cont'd.**

CMV peptides, the QuantiFERON-CMV (Cellestis Ltd., Melbourne, Australia).[14] This commercial assay is simpler to perform than the tetramer-based approach for quantification and functional analysis of antigen-specific CD8 T cells. It has been applied in the context of risk prediction for CMV in organ transplant and allogeneic hematopoietic cell transplant (HCT) patients. However, this assay has theoretical limitations in that assessing the production of a single cytokine is unlikely to represent the breadth of the immune response to a complex specific antigen such as CMV.

ACTIVATION AND FUNCTION OF NK CELLS

NK cells are innate immune lymphocytes that provide the cellular basis for innate responses to specific viruses and to tumor cells.[15−17] Unlike T and B cells of the adaptive immune system, NK cells do not have antigen-specific recognition and killing of target cells. NK cells participate directly in effector functions via cytotoxicity and production of cytokines (*e.g.*, IFN-γ) upon activation. Proinflammatory cytokines such as IL-12, IL-15, and IL-18 trigger NK cell proliferation as well as cytotoxicity and production of IFN-γ.[18] The negative regulation of NK cells is controlled by receptors that recognize MHC class I molecules preventing NK cell—mediated cytotoxicity. In contrast, virally infected or tumor cells typically downregulate MHC class I, making them appropriate targets of NK cell—mediated cytotoxicity in the presence of relevant ligands expressed by the target cell. NK cells, like cytotoxic T cells,[19] contain granules with cytotoxic proteins including perforin and granzymes, which are serine proteases that recognize different substrates.

NK CELL CYTOTOXICITY

The majority of NK cells can be identified by a lack of CD3 on the cell surface in conjunction with the expression of CD56 (NCAM [neural cell adhesion molecule]) and CD16 (FcγRIII). NK cells can be subdivided into two major subsets based on their relative expression of CD56 and CD16: CD16$^{+++(\text{bright})}$ CD56$^{+/-(\text{dim})}$ NK cells, referred to as cytotoxic NK cells, and CD56$^{+++(\text{bright})}$ CD16 or CD16$^{+/-}$ NK cells, known as regulatory or cytokine-producing NK cells (Fig. 3.8). The majority (~90%) of circulating human NK cells belong to the cytotoxic category, while a minority (10%) represent cytokine-producing NK cells. Cytotoxicity can be subdivided into natural or spontaneous cytotoxicity directed largely toward virally infected cells or tumor cells, in the absence of prior stimulation or immunization, and antibody-dependent cellular cytotoxicity directed against antibody-coated target cells. NK cells go through a process of education or "licensing" whereby NK cells that express inhibitory receptors to self-MHC class I

molecules are called licensed, which means they are more functionally responsive to stimulation, whereas unlicensed NK cells lack receptors for self-MHC class I and are hyporesponsive (Fig. 3.9).

NK cell function is measured in the clinical laboratory by assessment of spontaneous (natural) NK cell cytotoxicity using an MHC class I–deficient myelogenous leukemia cell line, K562. Traditional methods for measuring NK cell cytotoxicity are similar to those used for assessing cytotoxic T cell (CTL) function based on varying effector:target ratios in a 4- to 16-hr ^{51}Cr-release assay compared with the no-lysis and 100% lysis conditions as described for the T-cell cytotoxicity assay. However, there is interest in the use of flow cytometry to measure spontaneous or IL-2-activated (lymphokine-activated killer [LAK]) NK cell cytotoxicity in the clinical laboratory to avoid radioactivity. One flow cytometric assay employed in the clinical laboratory involves the use of fluorescently labeled (Cell Tracker® dyes) target cells (K562) incubated with effector cells (donor or patient PBMC) in

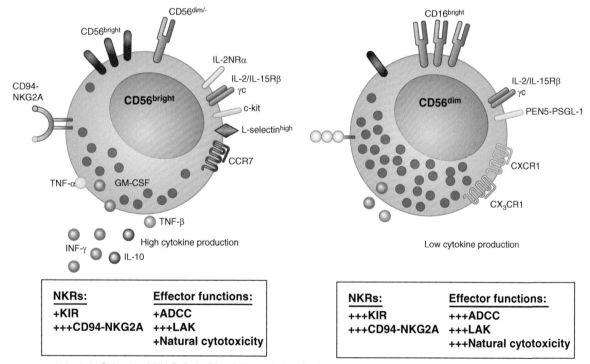

FIG. 3.8 Subsets of NK Cells in Blood. Natural killer (NK) cells are present as two major subsets in blood: cytotoxic NK cells (CD16^{++}CD56$^{+/-}$) and cytokine-producing NK cells (CD56^{++}). The former accounts for 90% of NK cells in circulation and the latter, 10%. The cytotoxic NK cells are very efficient in mediating target cell killing via spontaneous (natural), lymphokine-activated (LAK), or antibody-dependent cytotoxicity mechanisms. (Adapted from figure in Cooper MA, et al. *Trends Immunol* 2001;22:633–40.)

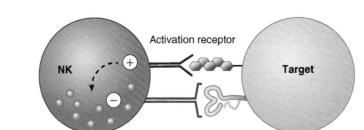

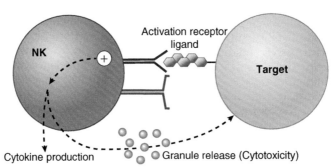

FIG. 3.9 Target Recognition by Natural Killer Cells for Cytotoxic Function. NK cells have inhibitory receptors for self—major histocompatibility complex (MHC) class I. Therefore NK cells do not kill target cells expressing MHC class I (upper panel). However, when MHC class I expression is downregulated (viral infections, tumors), the target cell is primed for NK cell cytotoxicity, which is mediated by granule exocytosis and release of cytotoxic proteins, including perforin and granzymes (lower panel). (Adapted from figure in French AR and Yokoyama WM. *Arthritis Res Ther* 2004;6:8–14.)

the absence (spontaneous) or presence of IL-2 (LAK). Following coincubation, the lysis of target cells is measured by using 7-AAD (7-amino-actinomycin-D) (Fig. 3.10). IL-2 enhances cytotoxic function with increased lytic potential against a broad range of target cells. IL-2 also induces IFN-γ secretion by NK cells with upregulation of activation markers, such as CD25 and CD69.[20] Treg cells control NK cell activation and cytotoxic function by limiting access to IL-2.[21] Other methods for measuring NK cell cytotoxic function that are primarily used in the research setting include the use of image cytometry,[22] microchip screening,[23] and flow-based assays using other dyes, such as calcein AM.[24]

The direct measurement of NK cell cytotoxic function is useful in a variety of clinical contexts, especially in patients with inherited immune defects affecting NK cells and function, including but not limited to recurrent/persistent herpesvirus infections and familial/primary hemophagocytic lymphohistiocytosis (FLH/HLH). There are other parameters that are widely used as surrogates of cytotoxicity, including flow cytometric measurement of granule exocytosis/

degranulation. The membrane of cytotoxic granules in both NK cells and CD8 T cells is composed of several proteins, including CD107a (lysosomal-associated membrane protein 1 [LAMP-1]). On stimulation of NK cells and CD8 cytotoxic T cells, CD107a is upregulated and expressed on the cell surface (Fig. 3.11) concomitantly with cytokine secretion and target cell lysis and therefore has been frequently used to extrapolate the magnitude of cytotoxic activity.[25,26] Degranulation (CD107a expression) assays have gained traction in the assessment of FHL.[27] The exception is in patients with mutations in the gene encoding perforin (*PRF1*; FHL type 2) where degranulation (CD107a expression) of cytotoxic cells is normal while cytotoxicity is abnormal. Therefore while degranulation assays may provide relevant information, they cannot substitute for direct measurement of cytotoxicity in all settings (Fig. 3.10B).

NK cells also mediate killing of target cells, via recognition of surface-bound immunoglobulin through the Fcγ receptors (Ig-Fc receptors, specifically CD16 or FcγRIIIa), through a mechanism called antibody-dependent cellular cytotoxicity (ADCC). ADCC has

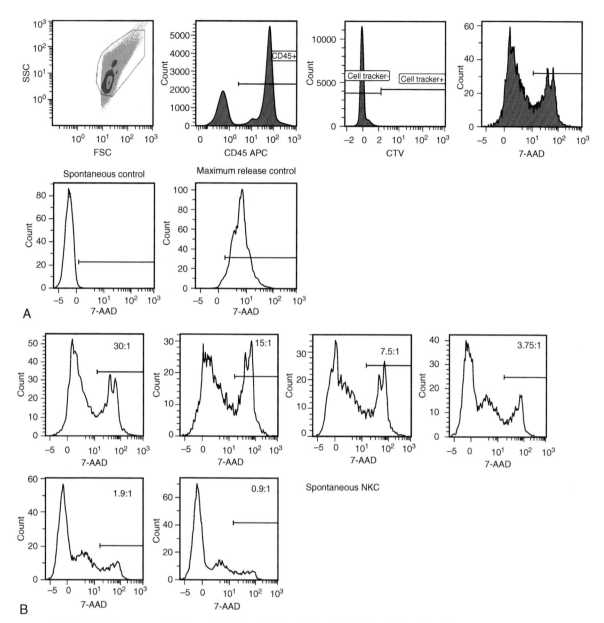

FIG. 3.10 Assessment by Flow Cytometry of Natural Killer Cell Cytotoxic Function. The "gold standard" for measuring natural killer cell cytotoxicity (NKC) uses a radioactive label for target cells. In the flow-based assay, target cells (K562, a major histocompatibility complex [MHC] class I–negative erythroleukemia cell line derived from a patient with chronic myelogenous leukemia [CML] in blast crisis) are labeled with a fluorescent marker, Cell Tracker® (CTV). A The gating strategy for analysis is shown. Peripheral blood mononuclear cells (PBMCs) from healthy controls or patients are cocultured with labeled target cells, and the two cell populations are identified by forward scatter (FSC) and side scatter (SSC) parameters. Afterward, CD45$^+$ lymphocytes are identified because NK cells (effector cells) are within the lymphocyte subset. CTV$^+$ and CTV$^-$ cells are separated; CTV$^+$ cells that are also 7-amino-actinomycin-D (7-AAD)$^+$ are identified as killed target cells, and their frequency is estimated. A negative control for spontaneous cytotoxicity is achieved by incubation of labeled target cells without effector cells added (called spontaneous control). A positive control for maximal cytotoxicity is achieved by incubating labeled target cells for the same duration but using a permeabilization/fixation method to obtain maximal cell death and fluorescent-positive cells (called maximum release control). B depicts spontaneous NK cell cytotoxicity with different concentrations of effector cells (PBMC; E) to a single concentration of target cells (T) starting at 30:1. The data are expressed as delta (Δ)% cytotoxicity after the spontaneous control signal is subtracted from the E:T signal for each concentration.

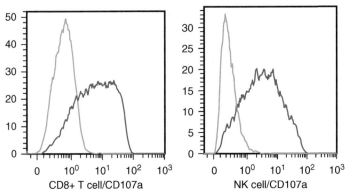

FIG. 3.11 Measurement of Cellular Degranulation. Cytotoxic lymphocytes undergo degranulation upon stimulation before mediating cytotoxic function. As a result of the degranulation process, CD107a, expressed intracellularly, is now expressed on the cell surface and can be assessed by flow cytometry. Degranulation can be determined in the CD8[+] T cells (left panel) and natural killer (NK) cells (right panel). In this analysis, peripheral blood mononuclear cells (PBMCs) were stimulated with phorbol myristate acetate (PMA) (10 ng/mL) and ionomycin (1 μg/mL) for 3 hours. Following stimulation, cells were stained for CD107a in CD8[+] T cells (left panel) and in NK cells (right panel). NK cells can also be stimulated with K562 cells as an alternative to mitogen stimulation. The degranulation assay is frequently used as a surrogate for, or as an adjunct to, measurement of cellular cytotoxicity.

also traditionally used the ^{51}Cr method discussed above, although currently flow cytometry has largely replaced radioactive methods. ADCC assays are particularly relevant in the assessment of antitumor responses, especially of new biological immunomodulatory agents, and of the function of alloantibodies in allograft rejection. Recently a method for assessing ADCC by flow cytometry using cryopreserved PBMC has been described,[28] although most clinical laboratories use fresh samples in these functional assays.

ASSESSMENT OF REGULATORY T-CELL FUNCTION

Regulatory T cells (FOXP3[+]Treg) have been well described over the past several years as a distinct subset of T cells that are both developmentally and functionally unique and essential to maintaining immune homeostasis and self-tolerance.[29,30] The major subpopulations of Treg cells include natural Treg (nTreg) cells that are produced in the thymus and induced Treg (iTreg) cells that are generated in the periphery from conventional FOXP3[-]CD4[+] T cells.[31] The dysfunction of Treg cells results in severe autoimmunity, with IPEX serving as the classic prototype.[3,32] Besides their role in controlling development of autoimmunity, lack of Treg cells or abnormal Treg function has been implicated in the etiopathogenesis of graft-versus-host disease (GVHD)[33] and

allograft rejection, while its presence and normal function have been shown to promote allograft tolerance in solid-organ transplantation.[34,35]

Key Concepts
Regulatory T Cells and B Cells

- Regulatory T cells (Tregs) and B cells (Bregs) are distinct subsets of cells with immune regulatory potential and importance in maintaining immune homeostasis and self-tolerance, preventing autoimmunity, and limiting inflammatory damage.
- FOXP3 transcription factor is a marker for natural regulatory T cells; while there are no specific cellular markers that define Breg, production of interleukin (IL)-10 is considered a hallmark.
- Both Treg and Breg have been shown to play important roles in autoimmunity, in graft-versus-host disease (GVHD), and in mediating transplant tolerance.
- Treg function is measured *in vitro* through different types of suppression assays, while Bregs are characterized by their ability to produce IL-10 when stimulated via toll-like receptor (TLR9)/B-cell receptor (BCR) or CD40L cross-linking.
- Natural, thymic-derived Tregs are CD4[+]25[+]FOXP3[+] while Bregs are CD19[+]CD24[hi]CD38[hi]IL-10[+].
- Treg can also be induced in the periphery from conventional T cells through cytokine signals (iTreg).

Treg cell function is measured *in vitro* with Treg suppression assays, which utilize sorted CD4$^+$CD25$^+$ Treg cells in a coculture system with conventional effector T cells to assess suppression of proliferation.[36] However, there are limitations to this approach, including the issue of whether the Treg suppression assays *in vitro* reflect the biological process *in vivo*. In addition, antigen-specific Treg suppression cannot be adequately assessed due to the technical difficulties in obtaining sufficient numbers of antigen-specific cells, so the use of a polyclonal activation model with bulk PBMC represents the standard to study Treg suppression. Rapid tests for Treg cell function have been described using short-term (7–20 hr) flow-based assays to measure suppression of T-cell activation marker expression (CD40L and CD69). These assays utilize effector T cells (CD4$^+$25$^-$) activated with anti-CD3/anti-CD28 beads with and without the addition of freshly isolated Treg cells or *ex vivo* expanded Treg cells.[37,38] When implementing Treg suppression assays in the clinical diagnostic laboratory, a number of technical considerations can confound the interpretation of results, and these are well described by McMurchy et al.[39] Also, it remains unclear whether standard *in vitro* Treg suppression assays can adequately account for the significant complexity of Treg subsets that may have different functional properties in various clinical contexts. Therefore the newer techniques of mass cytometry may be required to address the phenotypic diversity[40] and to eventually be harnessed either to evolving applications or other technology to analyze the functional complexity of these populations.

DETERMINATION OF SIGNALING AND DNA REPAIR PATHWAYS IN LYMPHOCYTES VIA PHOSPHOFLOW CYTOMETRY

A key aspect of studying lymphocyte responses is to assess signaling in appropriate lymphocyte subsets and its alteration in pathological conditions. A versatile tool called phosphoflow is unique in its ability to allow the study of multiple intracellular signaling molecules in specific lymphocyte populations at a single-cell level.[41] Phosphoflow assays for the signal transducer and activator of transcription (STAT) molecules (Fig. 3.12) have been well described.[42,43] The use of phosphoflow assays to assess Bruton's tyrosine kinase (BTK) phosphorylation in X-linked agammaglobulinemia (XLA) with leaky (hypomorphic) defects as well

as to assess radiosensitivity and the DNA repair pathway will be covered briefly.

Key Concepts
Assessment of DNA Repair Pathways by Phosphoflow

- DNA double-strand break (DSB) repair defects are relevant to VDJ recombination, isotype class switching, and lymphocyte maturation.
- Defects in this process can lead to immunodeficiency with susceptibility to infection and malignancy.
- Homologous recombination (HR), which is error-free, involves RAD50, RAD51, RAD52, and Mre11, while nonhomologous end-joining (NHEJ) is error-prone and utilizes Ku70/80, DNA-PKcs, Artemis, DNA Ligase IV, XRCC4, XLF/Cernunnos.
- ATM is a key regulator of cell-cycle checkpoints following irradiation-induced DSB and coordinates timing of phosphorylation of checkpoint proteins.
- Cell cycle analysis can help identify checkpoint defects and can be easily assessed by flow cytometry.
- Phosphorylation of H2AX (γH2AX) is a useful marker of DNA damage related to irradiation-induced DSB.
- However, several kinases phosphorylate H2AX, which can confound identification of specific defects; therefore assessing multiple proteins in the pathway allows identification of a broader group of DNA repair defects.
- Measurement of 53BP1 phosphorylation is a useful surrogate marker of the integrity of the chromatin ubiquitin ligase pathway.

Mutations in *BTK* impair B-cell maturation and function, and patients with XLA can have either no peripheral B cells (null mutations) or reduced B cells (hypomorphic/leaky mutations), depending on the specific genetic defect. Two regulatory tyrosine residues in BTK undergo rapid phosphorylation upon B-cell receptor (BCR) cross-linking (Y551 within the SH1 domain and Y223 in the SH3 domain).[44] Y551 is transphosphorylated by Src family kinases whereas Y223 is autophosphorylated. Phospho-BTK accounts for a small fraction (<5%) of the total BTK pool in BCR-activated B cells. BTK molecules are singly or doubly tyrosine-phosphorylated, and Y551 phosphorylation increases BTK activity, whereas Y223 phosphorylation is likely more relevant for protein-protein interactions due to its presence in the SH3 domain. Since the phosphorylation events are sequential (Y551 before Y223), the

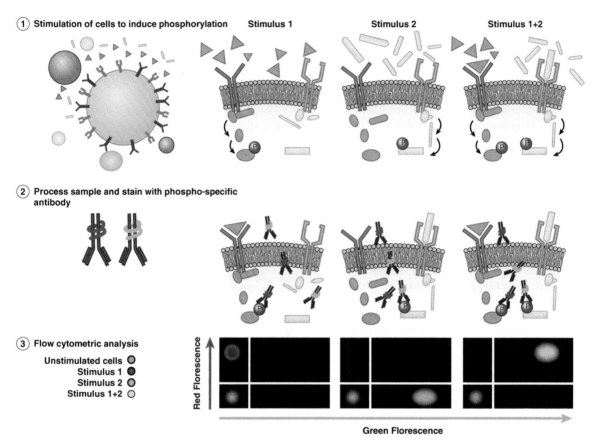

FIG. 3.12 Flow Cytometric Analysis of Cellular Phosphoproteins. Cells activated by specific stimuli can be assessed for activation and induction of specific signaling pathways by measuring phosphoproteins: A single stimulus or multiple stimuli can be used to phosphorylate different proteins, and intracellular staining can be performed with phospho-specific antibodies, which is subsequently analyzed by multicolor flow cytometry. See text for detailed explanation. (Figure modified from Figure 2 by Krutzik PO, et al. *Clin Immunol* 2004;110: 206–21.)

dephosphorylation event is also successive in the same order. In the flow assay, Y223 phosphorylation is measured after an anti-IgM antibody is used to cross-link the BCR (for 3 minutes) because Y551 phosphorylation could not be detected in the time interval the assay was performed. In addition to PBMC, Ramos cell line (a B-cell line derived from a patient with Burkitt lymphoma) is used as a control for B cells, while pervanadate (complex of vanadate with hydrogen peroxide), an irreversible protein tyrosine-phosphatase inhibitor, is used in this assay as a positive control (Fig. 3.13). In the Ramos cell line, it is possible to visualize the Y551 phosphorylation (Fig. 3.13) with pervanadate treatment.

A number of genetic disorders, collectively classified as XCIND (x-ray [irradiation] sensitivity, cancer susceptibility, immunodeficiency, neurological involvement, and double-strand DNA breakage), cause impairment in cellular ability to repair DNA double-strand breaks (DSB). These defects have a significant impact on the ability of cells to grow, differentiate, and function normally; they include ataxia telangiectasia (AT) due to *ATM* gene mutations and radiosensitive severe combined immunodeficiencies (rs-SCIDs) due to mutations in the *DCLRE1C*, *LIG4*, *NHEJ1*, and *PRKDC* genes. These disorders make it very desirable to have an assay capable of rapidly assessing DNA repair in lymphocytes in response to radiation damage. A flow

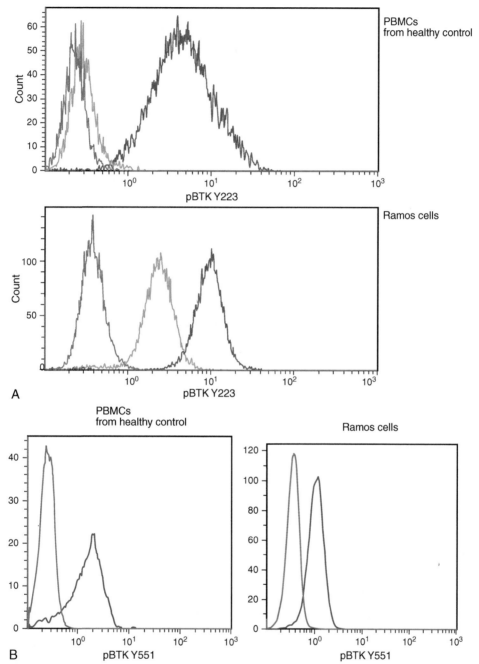

FIG. 3.13 Determination of BTK Phosphorylation in PBMC and Ramos B-Cell Line. Bruton's tyrosine kinase (BTK) phosphorylation can be assessed in B cells in X-linked agammaglobulinemia (XLA) patients with leaky defects who have some preserved B cells in blood. A B cells are stimulated with either anti-immunoglobulin M (IgM) (B-cell receptor [BCR] cross-linking; green line) or pervanadate (positive control; red line). The example shown here is for BTK phosphorylation at the Y223 residue in peripheral blood mononuclear cells (PBMCs) from a healthy donor (top panel) and a B-cell line, Ramos cells (bottom panel). The blue line represents the unstimulated control. B BTK phosphorylation of the Y551 residue is shown for PBMCs from a healthy donor (left) and Ramos cells (right). The phosphorylation of the Y551 residue cannot be visualized for anti-IgM stimulation, and therefore data are shown only for the positive control, pervanadate.

cytometry assay has been developed that is capable of measuring the function of several proteins in the DNA repair pathway after induction of DSBs via irradiation (Fig. 3.14). The assay includes assessment of nonphosphorylated ATM protein and 53BP1[45,46] without irradiation to determine the amount of native protein present. Following low-dose irradiation, the function of ATM and ATR (ATM-Rad3-related kinase) pathways is assessed by analyzing the autophosphorylation of ATM at serine 1981. This step is required for ATM activation and is followed by phosphorylation of downstream targets SMC1, H2AX, 53BP1, and CHK1. H2AX is a histone that belongs to the H2A family and is a component of the histone octamer in nucleosomes. It is phosphorylated by both ATM and ATR and is the first step in the recruitment and localization of DNA repair proteins.[47] In patients with AT, there is a complete absence of phosphorylation of ATM, SMC1, and 53BP1 after irradiation-induced DSBs. Phosphorylation of H2AX appears normal, as it is also phosphorylated by ATR; however, the magnitude of phosphorylation is significantly decreased (Fig. 3.15). The kinetics of phosphorylation indicates that maximal phosphorylation occurs 1 hr after induction of DSB and that there is dephosphorylation by 24 hr postirradiation (not shown). This flow-based assay enables a rapid assessment of radiation sensitivity as well as the ability to visualize the function of multiple proteins of the DNA repair pathway. It can also be used to characterize the DNA repair function of known and unknown genetic defects, and it can identify functional phenotypes in patients with atypical presentations that may be missed if only genetic information is used.

ANALYSIS OF B-CELL FUNCTION

While T cells and NK cells form the foundation of the cellular immune response, B cells are the main driver of humoral immunity. B cells are multifaceted in their function; they produce antibodies via differentiation into plasma cells, act as APCs for T cells, and secrete potent immunomodulatory cytokines while downregulating immune responses via IL-10 production. B cells can proliferate in response to polyclonal mitogenic stimuli such as PWM (Fig. 3.16), albeit with a much weaker response than seen with T cells stimulated with PHA (Fig. 3.3). Clearly, the starting point for any evaluation of B-cell function involves measuring serum immunoglobulin levels followed by *in vivo* antibody responses to vaccination with both protein (*e.g.*, tetanus toxoid) and carbohydrate (*e.g.*, Pneumovax 23) antigens.[48]

A more recent area of focus in laboratory evaluation of B cells has been the regulatory function of B cells, specifically with regard to the subset classified as regulatory B (Breg) cells. B cells that secrete IL-10 have been described as Breg cells and are now recognized to be an important component of the host immune response that protects against autoimmunity and also limits inflammatory damage.[49–51] In humans, the phenotype of Breg cells has been described as CD19+CD27−CD24hiCD38hiCD5+CD1dhi. However, the ability to produce IL-10 appears to be the defining feature rather than any particular constellation of cell-surface markers.[52] Also, unlike Treg cells, no exclusive transcription factor equivalent to FOXP3 is expressed in Breg cells. In general, IL-10+ Breg cells in blood and spleen appear to be enriched in the CD19+CD27+CD24hi memory B-cell subset. IL-10 exerts potent antiinflammatory effects and enhances survival, proliferation, differentiation, and isotype class-switching of B cells. Both naïve and memory human B cells have the ability to produce IL-10 in response to stimulation via TLR9 and the BCR, but only ∼15% of B cells can produce IL-10 in response to stimulation. Stimulation through CD40L or IL-21 also promotes differentiation of IL-10-producing Breg cells. CD19+CD24hiCD38hi Breg cells play critical regulatory roles in autoimmune disease, chronic GvHD, and transplant tolerance.[53–55]

In the diagnostic laboratory, Breg cells can be assessed by isolating PBMC from blood and culturing with CpG-B (TLR9 stimulation) or CpG-B plus recombinant CD40L for 3 days *in vitro*, followed by the addition of PMA, ionomycin, and brefeldin A (BFA) for the last 5 hours of culture. Cells can then be harvested, washed, and stained with CD19 and IL-10 antibodies (the latter requires intracellular staining) and then analyzed with a flow cytometer. To assess the presence of Breg cells in blood without *in vitro* differentiation, blood or PBMC can be analyzed for CD19+CD24hiCD38hi B cells that are positive for intracellular IL-10 using a similar flow cytometry protocol, but the levels of these cells can be highly variable, and accuracy of detection and quantitation is likely to be dependent on the analytical method and clinical context.*

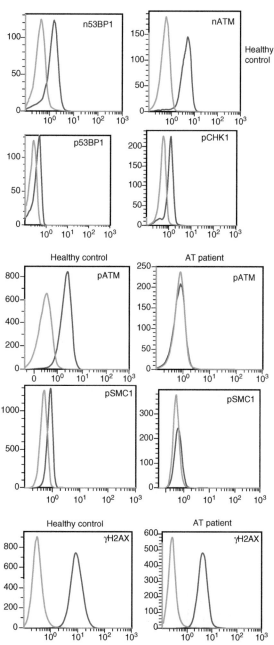

FIG. 3.14 Analysis of Radiosensitivity in Lymphocytes by Flow Cytometry. DNA repair pathway defects can be rapidly and sensitively analyzed by flow cytometry. The top panels show expression of native (nonphosphorylated) 53BP1 (n53BP1) and ATM (nATM) proteins and phosphorylated (p) 53BP1 (p53BP1) and CHK1 (pCHK1) proteins in total lymphocytes. The lower panels demonstrate normal ATM auto-phosphorylation in T cells of a healthy donor and absent (abnormal) phosphorylation of ATM (pATM) in T cells of a patient with ataxia telangiectasia (AT) on exposure to low-dose (2 Gy) radiation. The green line represents the unirradiated sample, and the red line represents the data postirradiation. AT patients also show an inability of ATM to phosphorylate downstream targets, such as SMC1 (pSMC1) in T cells. This is also true for other lymphocyte subsets (B cells and natural killer [NK] cells). Histone H2AX is phosphorylated (γH2AX) as a result of DNA double-strand breaks (DSBs) from exposure to radiation. No defect is apparent in γH2AX in AT when assessing the frequency of cells that express γH2AX.

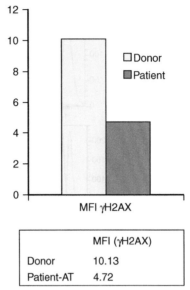

	MFI (γH2AX)
Donor	10.13
Patient-AT	4.72

FIG. 3.15 The Usefulness of Assessing Mean Fluorescence Intensity for Flow-Based Radiation Sensitivity Analyses. Mean fluorescence intensity (MFI) can provide additional valuable information on DNA repair defects and should be used along with frequency analysis, as demonstrated in Fig. 3.14. In ataxia telangiectasia (AT) patients, although the proportion of γH2AX appears normal, it is significantly decreased (by >50% in AT (purple bar) compared with healthy controls (blue bar).

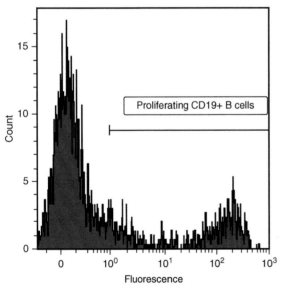

FIG. 3.16 Evaluation of B-Cell Function by Measuring Proliferation to Mitogen. B cells can proliferate on stimulation with certain mitogens, similar to T cells. B cells do not respond well to phytohemagglutinin (PHA) but can proliferate *in vitro* on stimulation with pokeweed mitogen (PWM), although it is a relatively weak B-cell stimulant. B-cell proliferation can be assessed by flow-based proliferation in CD19^{+} B cells.

SUMMARY

On the Horizon

- The advent of newer assays, including flow cytometry based as described herein, are likely to replace traditional and often less sensitive radioactive or other cumbersome methods for assessing lymphocyte function.
- Microchip and advanced mass cytometry techniques, along with imaging cytometry, may offer newer, multiplex approaches to the assessment of lymphocyte subsets, individually and in cellular interactions.
- Functional and phenotypic data need to be ideally correlated with relevant genomic, transcriptomic, proteomic, metabolomic, epigenomic, and microbiome analyses for effective characterization of the complex interactions that govern the immune response in the normal and dysregulated state.
- This will necessitate further refinements of "big data" analysis, which can include, but is not limited to, experimental studies in addition to computational modeling. Examples include antigen-specific characterization of individual B-cell and T-cell receptors in an individual as an extension of current "deep-sequencing" repertoire analysis or transcriptomic analysis during immune quiescence or activation on a multidimensional scale.

In conclusion, lymphocyte responses in humans can be assessed using a variety of analytical tools as described in this chapter and applied to many clinical contexts, including but not limited to primary immunodeficiencies, autoimmunity, transplantation, and immune dysregulation disorders. Most of these measurements use cells from blood and not from other lymphoid tissues due to accessibility and ease of generating control reference ranges. This chapter is not an exhaustive treatise on all aspects of lymphocyte function and the immune response, nor does it cover all areas of normal and abnormal pathology in this context. Rather, it is meant to take the reader on a tour of the immune landscape and to provide salient highlights of the diversity and relevance of lymphocyte function.

REFERENCES

1. Puga I, Cols M, Barra CM, et al. B cell-helper neutrophils stimulate the diversification and production of immunoglobulin in the marginal zone of the spleen. *Nat Immunol.* 2012;13(2):170–180.
2. Vinuesa CG, Chang PP. Innate B cell helpers reveal novel types of antibody responses. *Nat Immunol.* 2013;14(2):119–126.
3. Torgerson TR, Ochs HD. Immune dysregulation, polyendocrinopathy, enteropathy, X-linked: forkhead box protein 3 mutations and lack of regulatory T cells. *J Allergy Clin Immunol.* 2007;120(4):744–750, quiz 51–2.
4. Sakaguchi S, Wing K, Onishi Y, et al. Regulatory T cells: how do they suppress immune responses? *Int Immunol.* 2009;21(10):1105–1111.
5. Long EO, Kim HS, Liu D, et al. Controlling natural killer cell responses: integration of signals for activation and inhibition. *Annu Rev Immunol.* 2013;31:227–258.
6. Buck MD, O'Sullivan D, Pearce EL. T cell metabolism drives immunity. *J Exp Med.* 2015;212(9):1345–1360.
7. Wherry EJ, Kurachi M. Molecular and cellular insights into T cell exhaustion. *Nat Rev Immunol.* 2015;15(8):486–499.
8. Abraham RS. Lymphocyte activation. In: Detrick B, Schmitz JL, Hamilton RG, eds. *Manual of Molecular and Clinical Laboratory Immunology.* 8th ed. Washington, DC: ASM Press; 2016:269–279.
9. Abraham RS, Aubert G. Flow cytometry, a versatile tool for diagnosis and monitoring of primary immunodeficiencies. *Clin Vaccine Immunol.* 2016;23(4):254–271.
10. Appay V. The physiological role of cytotoxic CD4(+) T-cells: the holy grail? *Clin Exp Immunol.* 2004;138(1):10–13.
11. van Leeuwen EM, Remmerswaal EB, Heemskerk MH, et al. Strong selection of virus-specific cytotoxic CD4+ T-cell clones during primary human cytomegalovirus infection. *Blood.* 2006;108(9):3121–3127.
12. Snyder JE, Bowers WJ, Livingstone AM, et al. Measuring the frequency of mouse and human cytotoxic T cells by the Lysispot assay: independent regulation of cytokine secretion and short-term killing. *Nat Med.* 2003;9(2):231–235.
13. Mbitikon-Kobo FM, Bonneville M, Sekaly RP, et al. Ex vivo measurement of the cytotoxic capacity of human primary antigen-specific CD8 T cells. *J Immunol Methods.* 2012;375(1-2):252–257.
14. Walker S, Fazou C, Crough T, et al. Ex vivo monitoring of human cytomegalovirus-specific CD8+ T-cell responses using QuantiFERON-CMV. *Transpl Infect Dis.* 2007;9(2):165–170.
15. Colonna M, Jonjic S, Watzl C. Natural killer cells: fighting viruses and much more. *Nat Immunol.* 2011;12(2):107–110.
16. Vivier E, Raulet DH, Moretta A, et al. Innate or adaptive immunity? The example of natural killer cells. *Science.* 2011;331(6013):44–49.
17. Kreud AG, Mundy-Bosse BL, Yu J, et al. The broad spectrum of natural killer cell diversity. *Immunity.* 2017;47:820–833.
18. Chan CJ, Smyth MJ, Martinet L. Molecular mechanisms of natural killer cell activation in response to cellular stress. *Cell Death Differ.* 2014;21(1):5–14.
19. Sun JC, Lanier LL. NK cell development, homeostasis and function: parallels with CD8(+) T cells. *Nat Rev Immunol.* 2011;11(10):645–657.
20. Yu TK, Caudell EG, Smid C, et al. IL-2 activation of NK cells: involvement of MKK1/2/ERK but not p38 kinase pathway. *J Immunol.* 2000;164(12):6244–6251.
21. Gasteiger G, Hemmers S, Firth MA, et al. IL-2-dependent tuning of NK cell sensitivity for target cells is controlled by regulatory T cells. *J Exp Med.* 2013;210(6):1167–1178.
22. Somanchi SS, McCulley KJ, Somanchi A, et al. A novel method for assessment of natural killer cell cytotoxicity using image cytometry. *PLoS ONE.* 2015;10(10):e0141074.
23. Guldevall K, Brandt L, Forslund E, et al. Microchip screening platform for single cell assessment of NK cell cytotoxicity. *Front Immunol.* 2016;7:119.
24. Jang YY, Cho D, Kim SK, et al. An improved flow cytometry-based natural killer cytotoxicity assay involving calcein AM staining of effector cells. *Ann Clin Lab Sci.* 2012;42(1):42–49.
25. Alter G, Malenfant JM, Altfeld M. CD107a as a functional marker for the identification of natural killer cell activity. *J Immunol Methods.* 2004;294(1-2):15–22.
26. Betts MR, Brenchley JM, Price DA, et al. Sensitive and viable identification of antigen-specific CD8+ T cells by a flow cytometric assay for degranulation. *J Immunol Methods.* 2003;281(1-2):65–78.
27. Bryceson YT, Pende D, Maul-Pavicic A, et al. A prospective evaluation of degranulation assays in the rapid diagnosis of familial hemophagocytic syndromes. *Blood.* 2012;119(12):2754–2763.
28. Yamashita M, Kitano S, Aikawa H, et al. A novel method for evaluating antibody-dependent cell-mediated cytotoxicity by flowcytometry using cryopreserved human peripheral blood mononuclear cells. *Sci Rep.* 2016;6:19772.
29. Ohkura N, Kitagawa Y, Sakaguchi S. Development and maintenance of regulatory T cells. *Immunity.* 2013;38(3):414–423.

30. Sakaguchi S, Miyara M, Costantino CM, et al. FOXP3+ regulatory T cells in the human immune system. *Nat Rev Immunol.* 2010;10(7):490−500.

31. Schmitt EG, Williams CB. Generation and function of induced regulatory T cells. *Front Immunol.* 2013;4:152.

32. Barzaghi F, Passerini L, Bacchetta R. Immune dysregulation, polyendocrinopathy, enteropathy, x-linked syndrome: a paradigm of immunodeficiency with autoimmunity. *Front Immunol.* 2012;3:211.

33. Beres AJ, Drobyski WR. The role of regulatory T cells in the biology of graft versus host disease. *Front Immunol.* 2013;4: 163.

34. Li XC, Turka LA. An update on regulatory T cells in transplant tolerance and rejection. *Nat Rev Nephrol.* 2010; 6(10):577−583.

35. Waldmann H, Hilbrands R, Howie D, et al. Harnessing FOXP3+ regulatory T cells for transplantation tolerance. *J Clin Invest.* 2014;124(4):1439−1445.

36. Boks MA, Zwaginga JJ, van Ham SM, et al. An optimized CFSE-based T-cell suppression assay to evaluate the suppressive capacity of regulatory T-cells induced by human tolerogenic dendritic cells. *Scand J Immunol.* 2010;72(2): 158−168.

37. Canavan JB, Afzali B, Scotta C, et al. A rapid diagnostic test for human regulatory T-cell function to enable regulatory T-cell therapy. *Blood.* 2012;119(8):e57−66.

38. Ruitenberg JJ, Boyce C, Hingorani R, et al. Rapid assessment of in vitro expanded human regulatory T cell function. *J Immunol Methods.* 2011;372(1-2):95−106.

39. McMurchy AN, Levings MK. Suppression assays with human T regulatory cells: a technical guide. *Eur J Immunol.* 2012;42(1):27−34.

40. Mason GM, Lowe K, Melchiotti R, et al. Phenotypic complexity of the human regulatory T cell compartment revealed by mass cytometry. *J Immunol.* 2015;195(5): 2030−2037.

41. Krutzik PO, Trejo A, Schulz KR, et al. Phospho flow cytometry methods for the analysis of kinase signaling in cell lines and primary human blood samples. *Methods Mol Biol.* 2011;699:179−202.

42. Fleisher TA, Dorman SE, Anderson JA, et al. Detection of intracellular phosphorylated STAT-1 by flow cytometry. *Clin Immunol.* 1999;90(3):425−430.

43. Murphy J, Goldberg GL. Flow cytometric analysis of STAT phosphorylation. *Methods Mol Biol.* 2013;967: 161−165.

44. Wahl MI, Fluckiger AC, Kato RM, et al. Phosphorylation of two regulatory tyrosine residues in the activation of Bruton's tyrosine kinase via alternative receptors. *Proc Natl Acad Sci USA.* 1997;94(21):11526−11533.

45. Panier S, Boulton SJ. Double-strand break repair: 53BP1 comes into focus. *Nat Rev Mol Cell Biol.* 2014;15(1):7−18.

46. Paull TT. Mechanisms of ATM Activation. *Annu Rev Biochem.* 2015;84:711−738.

47. Kuo LJ, Yang LX. Gamma-H2AX - a novel biomarker for DNA double-strand breaks. *Vivo.* 2008;22(3):305−309.

48. Abraham RS. Relevance of antibody testing in patients with recurrent infections. *J Allergy Clin Immunol.* 2012; 130(2):558−559, e6.

49. Mauri C, Bosma A. Immune regulatory function of B cells. *Annu Rev Immunol.* 2012;30:221−241.

50. Sarvaria A, Madrigal JA, Saudemont A. B cell regulation in cancer and anti-tumor immunity. *Cell Mol Immunol.* 2017; 14(8):662−674.

51. Rosser EC, Mauri C. Regulatory B cells: origin, phenotype, and function. *Immunity.* 2015;42(4):607−612.

52. Lin W, Cerny D, Chua E, et al. Human regulatory B cells combine phenotypic and genetic hallmarks with a distinct differentiation fate. *J Immunol.* 2014;193(5): 2258−2266.

53. Flores-Borja F, Bosma A, Ng D, et al. CD19+CD24 hiCD38hi B cells maintain regulatory T cells while limiting TH1 and TH17 differentiation. *Sci Transl Med.* 2013; 5(173):173ra23.

54. Nouel A, Simon Q, Jamin C, et al. Regulatory B cells: an exciting target for future therapeutics in transplantation. *Front Immunol.* 2014;5:11.

55. Sarantopoulos S, Blazar BR, Cutler C, et al. B cells in chronic graft-versus-host disease. *Biol Blood Marrow Transplant.* 2015;21(1):16−23.

CHAPTER 4

Evaluation of Neutrophil Function

DEBRA LONG PRIEL • DOUGLAS B. KUHNS

Neutrophils, also known as polymorphonuclear neutrophils (PMNs; because of their multilobed nucleus) or granulocytes (because of the numerous granules found in the cytoplasm), are major contributors to innate host defense against invading microorganisms, particularly bacteria and fungi. Neutrophils are bone marrow−derived, terminally differentiated cells that are incapable of further cellular division but may also be derived from progenitor populations in the spleen.[1] Early studies indicated that neutrophils have a short life span in the circulation ($t_{1/2}=$ 6−8 hours) and then survive an additional 1−2 days in the surrounding tissue[2]; more recent data suggest that neutrophils may survive 10 times longer in circulation, up to 5.4 days.[3]

Neutrophils, with a diameter of 10−15 μm and a volume of 346 μm³, have a unique morphology. The nucleus of the mature neutrophil is segmented into 3−5 lobes with chromosomes randomly distributed among the lobes. Neutrophils also have an extensive array of storage granules prepackaged with specific proteins defined by the differentiation stage during maturation.[4] Granules are classified into four distinct populations: azurophilic, specific, gelatinase, and secretory granules. Azurophilic granules contain myeloperoxidase, lysozyme, antimicrobial peptides, defensins, proteases, and the lysosomal acid hydrolases. The specific granules contain lactoferrin, lysozyme, and vitamin B_{12}−binding protein and also serve as storage pools for CD11b/CD18 and cytochrome b_{558} of the superoxide anion radical ($O_2^{\bullet-}$)−generating enzyme, nicotinamide adenine dinucleotide phosphate (NADPH) oxidase, or NOX2. The gelatinase granules are a subset of the specific granules that have a high content of gelatinase. The secretory granules are highly mobilizable intracellular vesicles that contain alkaline phosphatase and other surface antigens.

The primary function of neutrophils is the ingestion (phagocytosis) and subsequent killing of microorganisms. This process requires the assembly of NOX2, a multiphagocyte oxidase (phox) component enzyme complex consisting of at least three cytosolic components—$p47^{phox}$, $p67^{phox5}$, and $p40^{phox6}$—and two membrane components—$p22^{phox}$ and $gp91^{phox}$—that constitute cytochrome b_{558}.[7,8] This enzyme reduces molecular O_2 to $O_2^{\bullet-}$ using NADPH generated by the oxidation of glucose through the pentose phosphate pathway; $O_2^{\bullet-}$ either spontaneously or enzymatically converts to hydrogen peroxide (H_2O_2). In the presence of a metal, such as iron (Fe^{2+}), H_2O_2 and $O_2^{\bullet-}$ can react to form the highly reactive hydroxyl radical, $OH^{\bullet}$. Alternatively, the azurophilic granule constituent, myeloperoxidase, catalyzes the formation of hypochlorous acid from H_2O_2 and chloride (Cl^-). The combined activities of these reactive O_2 species (ROS), antimicrobial peptides, and lysosomal hydrolases result in the ultimate destruction of the ingested microorganism.[9] Excess production of ROS and release of lysosomal hydrolases into the extracellular milieu can lead to tissue damage and inflammation.[9]

Neutrophils can also contribute extracellular microbicidal activity through the formation of neutrophil extracellular traps (NETs), a matrix of DNA and granular enzymes that is purported to entrap bacteria and promote their killing.[10] During NET formation, the nucleus loses its lobular shape, the nuclear membrane disintegrates into a chain of vesicles surrounding the DNA, and granular integrity is lost. The nuclear material fills most of the cell, mixing with the granular contents. The cells round up and DNA is forcibly extruded from the cell, conveying with it granular enzymes trapped within the DNA matrix. Mitochondria in neutrophils are few in number and exhibit relatively little oxidative phosphorylation but may play an important role in NET formation. Activation of neutrophils by immune complexes results in marked depolarization of the mitochondria, increased mitochondrial ROS production, and redistribution of the mitochondria to the periphery of the neutrophil. A low-density subset of neutrophils may be more prone to NET formation.[11]

Core Laboratory Technologies in Clinical Immunology. https://doi.org/10.1016/B978-0-323-66149-2.00004-9

Neutrophils display a diverse array of cellular functions. Abnormalities in these functions can severely compromise host defense, leading to recurrent bacterial and fungal infections.[12] To localize specific deficiencies of neutrophil function, assays have been developed that mimic these functions both *in vivo* and *in vitro*. Often, a preliminary screening of several neutrophil functions is performed to localize deficits and then more vigorous testing of specific function is performed. Assays to assess neutrophil function should address several limitations—the number of cells required for the assay, the type of cell preparation needed (isolated neutrophils versus whole blood), the overall incubation time for the assay, the complexity of the assay, and the rapidity of data collection. These issues become more critical if multiple functional assays are planned concurrently. Since neutrophils cannot be stored or frozen and maintain viability, neutrophils from a normal subject are generally assayed in parallel to validate the results, doubling the number of assays to be performed. Additionally, isolation of neutrophils can take 1−2 hours, limiting the time available for functional assays. Fluorescent probes have increased the sensitivity of many of the assays and eliminated the need for radioactive probes. The use of multiwell microplates and microplate readers has reduced the number of cells required and has facilitated the collection of data. Experience in the handling of neutrophils and the time constraints of assays can limit the availability of this testing to laboratories that specialize in assessment of neutrophil function.

> **Key Concept**
> *Criteria to Assess Neutrophil Function*
>
> Because of (1) the time required to isolate neutrophils and (2) the shortened life span of neutrophils after isolation, assays of neutrophil function should have minimal complexity and enable rapid data collection.

NEUTROPHIL ISOLATION
Clinical Indications and Implications

Assays that avoid neutrophil isolation are preferred because of the artificial priming of neutrophils during isolation.[13] However, most assays require isolated neutrophils to eliminate any possible contributions of other leukocytes and blood components. In general, blood should be drawn using either citrate or heparin as anticoagulant and maintained at 20−25°C in polypropylene containers. Most isolation protocols require 1−2 hours to obtain purified neutrophils.

Principles and Interpretation of Laboratory Assessment

Most neutrophil isolation protocols use differences in the cell density as the basis for the separation. The relative densities of blood cells are as follows: erythrocytes > neutrophils and eosinophils > monocytes, lymphocytes, and basophils > platelets. Ficoll-Paque is a solution of sodium diatrizoate (a dense, triiodinated compound) and Ficoll (a polysaccharide) with a density (1.077 g/cc) that falls between the density of neutrophils and that of the mononuclear cells. To isolate neutrophils,[14] whole blood is diluted with saline and underlaid with Ficoll-Paque solution. After centrifugation for 30 minutes at 500 g, the less-dense monocytes, lymphocytes, basophils, and platelets remain at the upper interface of the Ficoll-Paque solution, whereas the denser erythrocytes and neutrophils pass through the solution and pellet at the bottom. The mononuclear cells are carefully harvested and the remaining Ficoll-Paque solution aspirated. The erythrocyte/neutrophil pellet is resuspended with saline and mixed with 3% dextran. Dextran promotes the formation of rouleaux by the erythrocytes, causing them to sediment more rapidly than the neutrophils at 1 g. The neutrophil-enriched supernatant fluid is harvested from the bulk of the erythrocytes. Contaminating erythrocytes are removed by a brief (30-second) hypotonic lysis with 0.2% saline. The isotonicity is quickly restored with an equal volume of 1.6% saline. A second hypotonic lysis removes many of the red blood cell (RBC) ghosts. In general, $1-2 \times 10^6$ neutrophils can be isolated per milliliter of whole blood from a normal subject with a normal white blood cell (WBC) count. All procedures are performed at room temperature, and the isolated cells are maintained in a balanced salt solution without divalent cations. The most common cell contaminants of the neutrophil preparation are eosinophils. Further purification of a standard neutrophil preparation with anti-CD16 magnetic immunobeads results in a neutrophil preparation that is generally ≥99% neutrophils. A second neutrophil isolation protocol that uses a discontinuous gradient of plasma/Percoll has often been used to minimize exposure of neutrophils to trace contamination by bacterial lipopolysaccharide (LPS) and reduce neutrophil priming.[15]

> **Key Concept**
> *Estimated Yield From Whole Blood*
>
> In general, $1-2 \times 10^6$ neutrophils can be isolated per milliliter of whole blood from a normal subject with a normal white blood cell count.

Isolated neutrophils are routinely frozen in aliquots of 5×10^6 cells/vial. For Western blot studies, neutrophils (1×10^6 cells/mL of buffer) are pretreated for 20 minutes with the cell permeant, irreversible serine protease inhibitor, diisopropylfluorophosphate (DFP, 1−5 mM). DFP is a volatile, potent neurotoxin that can irreversibly bind to and inactivate acetylcholinesterase and should be used with extreme caution. The cell suspension is then spun and the supernatant fluid removed from the cell pellet before freezing. Waste solutions and disposable laboratory items should be flushed with sodium hydroxide to inactivate any residual DFP. These frozen neutrophil pellets, though not viable, can also be a source of DNA for genetic analyses.

NEUTROPHIL HISTOCHEMICAL ANALYSIS
Clinical Indications and Implications
Because of their unique morphology, microscope examination of neutrophil preparations with a differential stain, such as Wright stain, or a histochemical stain, such as Kaplow stain, for myeloperoxidase[16] remains an essential element of neutrophil study and can provide valuable insight into some genetic immunodeficiencies.

Principle and Interpretation of Laboratory Assessment
In Wright's stain, the nucleus of a segmented neutrophil is normally multilobed (usually 2−5 lobes), and each lobe is connected by a narrow filament (Fig. 4.1A). The nuclear chromatin is coarsely clumped with purple staining. Nucleoli are generally not present. In a band neutrophil, the nucleus is horseshoe shaped, with no indication of constriction into lobes. The pink-violet staining of the cytosol is associated with numerous, evenly distributed, specific granules; occasionally a dark-staining primary granule may be present. Kaplow stain[16] identifies the myeloperoxidase-containing primary granules as dark blue granules uniformly distributed throughout the cytosol (Fig. 4.1B). Neutrophils (and platelets) from patients with Chédiak-Higashi syndrome have giant primary granules that are generally considered pathognomonic for the disease (see Fig. 4.1C).[17] Myeloperoxidase staining of Chédiak-Higashi neutrophils is very distinctive, with staining localized to the discrete giant primary granules (see Fig. 4.1D). Neutrophils from a patient with specific granule deficiency exhibit primarily bilobed nuclei (pseudo−Pelger-Huët anomaly) with a paucity of specific granule staining in the cytosol (see Fig. 4.1E).[18] Staining of the myeloperoxidase granules of neutrophils from a patient with specific granule deficiency appears normal, since the defect is primarily associated with the specific granules (see Fig. 4.1F). Neutrophils from a patient with myeloperoxidase deficiency fail to stain for myeloperoxidase in the neutrophils. However, the peroxidase in the eosinophilic granules continues to stain positive (see Fig. 4.1G).[19]

DETERMINATION OF GRANULE CONSTITUENTS
Clinical Indications and Implications
The granules of the neutrophils can be distinguished by their specific contents. Deficiency of only one granule constituent can be associated with a specific genetic defect, such as myeloperoxidase deficiency; alternatively, deficiency of multiple constituents of a certain granule can be associated with deficiency of an entire pool of granules, such as specific granule deficiency. Both enzymatic assays and immunoassays are available to determine the cellular content of many of these granule constituents.

Principles and Interpretation of Laboratory Assessment
The cellular content of neutrophils can be determined by solubilization of a neutrophil pellet with 0.2% Triton X-100, followed by sonication to disrupt the cells and generate a homogeneous lysate. Analysis of the lysate using commercial immunoassays can identify deficiencies of certain granule contents. Diagnosis of myeloperoxidase deficiency can be confirmed by analysis of neutrophil lysates. Similarly, deficiency of both lactoferrin and neutrophil gelatinase (matrix metalloprotein-9 [MMP-9]) is indicative of specific granule deficiency, although interestingly, specific granule deficiency is also associated with a deficiency of the α-defensins (human neutrophil peptides 1−3), stored in the azurophilic granules.[20]

ADHERENCE OF NEUTROPHILS
Clinical Indications and Implications
Adherence of neutrophils to the endothelium is a prerequisite step to the migration of neutrophils into the tissues. Neutrophils isolated from patients with leukocyte adhesion defect-1 (LAD-1) who lack the common β_2 integrin subunit CD18 exhibit abnormal adherence to the endothelium[21] and therefore are not able to migrate efficiently into the surrounding tissues, often resulting in marked granulocytosis.[22] LAD-2 is a milder form of the disease, in which patients exhibit a defect in fucose metabolism and glycoprotein biosynthesis.[23]

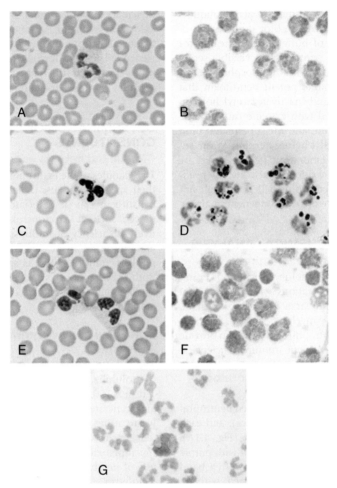

FIG. 4.1 Neutrophil Staining With Wright Stain and Kaplow Stain. (A, C, and E) Blood smears stained with Wright stain. (B, D, F, and G) Neutrophil preparations stained with Kaplow stain. (A, B) Neutrophils from a normal subject. (C, D) Neutrophils from a patient with Chédiak-Higashi syndrome. (E, F) Neutrophils from a patient with specific granule deficiency. (G) Neutrophils from a patient with myeloperoxidase deficiency. The blue positive-staining cell is an eosinophil.

Neutrophils from patients with LAD-2 exhibit abnormal expression of the glycoprotein L-selectin and fail to roll along the endothelium. However, they do exhibit normal β_2 integrin–mediated adherence.

Principles and Interpretation of Laboratory Assessment

Adherence of neutrophils can be assessed by measuring binding to plastic using a 96-well plate either uncoated or coated with fetal bovine serum or a specific extracellular matrix (ECM) protein, such as fibrinogen or fibronectin. Endothelial cell monolayers

harvested from human umbilical veins may serve as a more physiological substrate for the measurement of cell adhesion. Isolated neutrophils are preloaded with the cell permeant acetoxymethyl ester derivative of the fluorescent dye calcein (calcein-AM). Nonspecific esterases in the cytosol cleave the ester linkage, trapping the fluorescent probe in the cytosol. The labeled neutrophils are added to each well and incubated in the absence or presence of phorbol myristate acetate (PMA) to promote adherence through activation of the integrins. At the end of the incubation, the wells are washed three times to remove

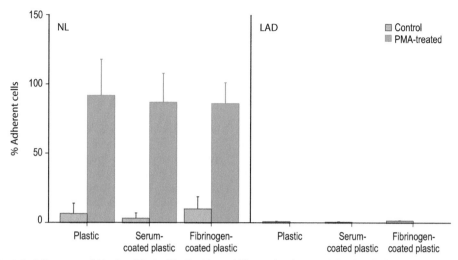

FIG. 4.2 Adherence of Neutrophils to Plastic: Normal Versus Leukocyte Adhesion Deficiency. Neutrophils (1×10^7 cells/mL in Hank's balanced salt solution [HBSS] without divalent cations) were preloaded with acetoxymethyl ester derivative of calcein (calcein-AM: 5 μg/mL) for 15 minutes at 37°C. The cells were washed twice and resuspended in HBSS/4-(2-hydroxyethyl)-1-piperazineethanesulfonic acid (HEPES) with 2% bovine serum albumin (BSA) at a cell concentration of 2×10^6/mL. The wells of a 96-well plate were coated for 1 hour at 37°C with 32 μL of either buffer alone, fetal bovine serum, or fibrinogen (2.5 mg/mL). The wells were washed three times, and then cells were added to each well (160 μL/well, 3.2×10^5/well). After a 10-minute preincubation at 37°C, PMA (100 ng/mL) was added and the plate was incubated for 30 minutes at 37°C. The wells were then washed three times with HBSS/HEPES to remove nonadherent neutrophils. The percentage of adherent cells was determined by the ratio of the fluorescence of the well compared with the fluorescence of a known standard well. The panel (NL) on the left represents the data (mean ± standard deviation [SD]) from 22 normal subjects and the panel on the right represents the data from three patients with leukocyte adhesion deficiency.

nonadherent cells. The fluorescence of each well is determined with a fluorescent microplate reader and compared with the fluorescence of a control well with a fixed number of fluorescent cells. As shown in the left panel of Fig. 4.2, under control conditions, fewer than 10% of the neutrophils adhere to plastic or to plastic coated with fetal bovine serum or fibrinogen. Treatment of normal neutrophils with PMA for 30 minutes results in the adherence of >90% of the neutrophils under all conditions. This adherence assay is valuable in the diagnosis of patients with leukocyte adhesion deficiency. As shown in the right panel of Fig. 4.2, neutrophils isolated from patients with LAD-1 generally exhibit <5% adherence under control conditions and do not increase adherence after treatment with PMA.

CHEMOTAXIS OF NEUTROPHILS

Clinical Indications and Implications

Neutrophil migration is a prerequisite for neutrophil accumulation at sites of inflammation. Patients with leukocyte chemotactic defects usually show recurrent skin abscesses and occasional life-threatening, invasive infections.

Principles and Interpretation of Laboratory Assessment

Chemotaxis *in vitro* is generally measured using a Boyden chamber. The Boyden chamber includes three components: a lower (chemoattractant) chamber, a nitrocellulose or polycarbonate filter layer, and an upper cell chamber. The lower compartments of the Boyden chamber are filled with a chemoattractant, such as formyl-methionyl-leucyl phenylalanine (fMLF; 10^{-8} M) or interleukin-8 (IL-8; 10^{-8} M). Alternatively, a rapid fluorescence-based measurement of neutrophil chemotaxis that uses a 96-well disposable chemotaxis chamber,[24] which can be read in a fluorescence microplate reader, can be used. The lower chamber contains the chemoattractant and is separated from the cellular compartment by a filter. However, instead of a top chamber, the filter has a hydrophobic mask around each filter site that creates surface tension in the cell suspension and aligns the suspension on the hydrophilic filter located directly above the chemoattractant chamber. Calcein-labeled neutrophils are placed on top of the filter. The chemotaxis chamber is incubated for up to 60 minutes at 37°C. Nonmigrating neutrophils atop the filter are rinsed off with buffer, and then the plate is read in a fluorescence microplate reader. The number of migrating neutrophils can be determined by comparison of the fluorescence to a standard well with a known number of fluorescent neutrophils. Less than 5×10^6 fluorescent neutrophils are needed to determine neutrophil chemotaxis using several doses of the chemoattractants, fMLF, IL-8, C5a, and leukotriene B_4. The advantages of this assay are high sensitivity, rapid acquisition and analysis of data, and reduced labor in loading the cell suspension. The 96-well format also allows for multiple comparisons to be made under identical conditions.

Instrumentation, such as the EZ-TAXIScan, is now available to monitor chemotaxis temporally. By acquiring digital images over time and analyzing them using imaging software, the coordinates of individual cells can be determined. Changes in the distance (and velocity) in the direction of the chemoattractant (directed migration) and orthogonal to the direction of the chemoattractant (random migration) can be determined. Tracks of multiple cells can be anchored at the origin and displayed graphically (Fig. 4.3, top

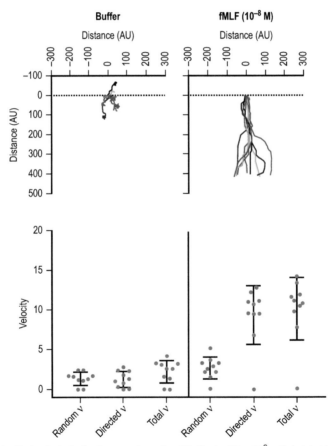

FIG. 4.3 Chemotactic Analysis. In the top panel, neutrophils (1 μL of 2×10^6 cells/mL in Hank's balanced salt solution [HBSS] with divalent cations) were added to the "Cell" well of EZ-TAXIScan and either buffer (left column) or formyl-methionyl-leucyl-phenylalanine (fMLF; 1×10^{-8} M, right column) was added to the "Chemoattractant" well. The cells were incubated for 60 minutes and images were collected every 2.5 minutes. Using the acquired images, 10 randomly chosen cells were electronically tracked and the paths of the cells plotted with their position at t = 0 anchored at the origin. Presented in the bottom panel are scattergrams of the average velocities of the individual cells that were tracked in the top panel.

panels). Adding time as a dimension in the analysis of chemotaxis provides a mechanism to evaluate simultaneously both chemotactic and chemokinetic responses in neutrophils and to detect more subtle defects. Using buffer as a chemoattractant, the average cellular velocity vector in the direction of the chemoattractant and the average cellular velocity vector orthogonal to the direction of the chemoattractant are typically equivalent (Fig. 4.3, bottom panel). When using a chemoattractant (e.g., fMLF, IL-8), typically there is marked increase in the average cellular velocity vector in the direction of the chemoattractant, but little change in the average cellular velocity vector orthogonal to the direction of the chemoattractant (see Fig. 4.3, bottom panel).

SURFACE ANTIGEN EXPRESSION
Clinical Indications and Implications
The expression of neutrophil membrane antigens is altered in vivo during exudation or after challenge with intravenous endotoxin. Flow cytometric analysis of adhesion molecules on the neutrophil cell surface can indirectly reflect neutrophil adhesion function. Patients with LAD-1 exhibit a deficit in the expression of the common β_2 integrin, CD18, resulting in deficiency in CD11a, CD11b, CD11c, and CD18.[25]

Principles and Interpretation of Laboratory Assessment
The expression of cell surface antigens is determined on neutrophils stained with specific fluorescent monoclonal antibodies (mAbs) and analyzed by flow cytometric analysis. Neutrophils stained with nonspecific isotype antibodies are used to determine the nonspecific background staining. To determine the expression of circulating neutrophils and avoid artifacts induced by neutrophil isolation, an aliquot of whole blood can be stained with the appropriate antibody before lysis of the erythrocytes. During flow cytometric analysis, the neutrophils are easily differentiated using their forward light scatter and right angle light scatter to gate on the neutrophil population. Since very little blood is needed (100 μL) for each antigen, neutrophils can be stained with a panel of antibodies to many relevant surface antigens so that a more complete representation of surface antigen expression on neutrophils can be obtained. The panel should include the β_2 integrins (CD11a, CD11b, CD11c, and CD18); selectins (CD62L); Fcγ receptors I, II, and III (CD64, CD32, and CD16); leukosialin (CD43); the common leukocyte antigen (CD45); and distinct surface markers for the granules—carcinoembryonic antigen-related cell

adhesion molecule 8 (CEACAM8, or CD66b), a GPI-anchored glycoprotein family member stored in the specific granules, and lysosomal-associated membrane protein 3 (LAMP-3, or CD63), stored in the azurophilic granules. During exudation, the expression of CD11b and CD18 is increased over that observed in peripheral neutrophils, whereas the expression of CD43 (leukosialin) and CD62L is markedly reduced.

The antibody 7D5 recognizes an extracellular epitope of gp91^{phox} and can be used to identify surface expression of gp91^{phox} and mobilization of latent pools of gp91^{phox} stored in the specific granules. Flow cytometric analysis of neutrophils stained with 7D5 can often be used to identify patients with X-linked chronic granulomatous disease (CGD) (no 7D5 staining) and X-linked chronic carriers of CGD (mosaic pattern of staining), particularly in patients where the number of cells available for testing is limited.

The expression of surface antigens can also be used to assess the responsiveness of neutrophils to particular ligands, such as fMLF and LPS. As shown in Fig. 4.4, neutrophils isolated from a patient who has a genetic defect in IL-1 receptor–associated kinase-4 (IRAK-4)[26] exhibit abnormal regulation of surface antigen expression to LPS but exhibit normal regulation of surface antigen expression to fMLF. Antigen expression can be upregulated because of translocation of latent antigen to the plasma membrane or downregulated because of either internalization or shedding of the antigen.

DEGRANULATION OF NEUTROPHILS
Clinical Indications and Implications
The proteases, acid hydrolases, and inflammatory mediators released from storage granules in the neutrophils can mediate bacterial killing, tissue damage, healing, and immune regulation. Lactoferrin that is released from specific granules can chelate iron, resulting in a bactericidal or bacteriostatic effect. Elevation of plasma lactoferrin is an indication of intravascular activation and degranulation of neutrophils.

Principles and Interpretation of Laboratory Assessment
Stimulation of neutrophils with various secretagogues can result in the release of granular enzymes into the extracellular fluid. Treatment of the neutrophils with cytochalasin b (5 μg/mL) disrupts microfilament assembly and facilitates the release of both specific and azurophilic enzymes. Since stimulation of neutrophil degranulation is often accompanied by ROS generation and oxidative inactivation of enzymes, both the cell

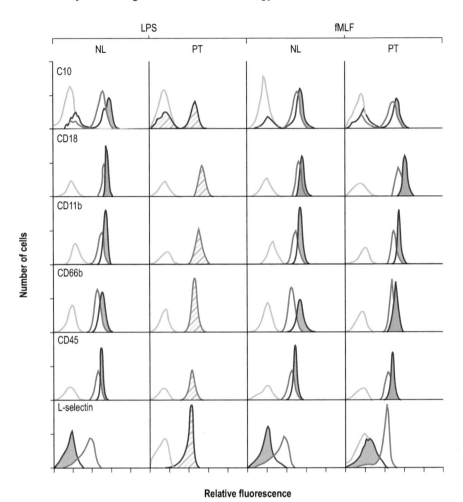

FIG. 4.4 Upregulation of Antigen Expression on Neutrophil Surfaces. Neutrophils (2.5 × 10^6/mL in Hank's balanced salt solution [HBSS] + 10% AB sera) isolated from a normal subject (NL) or from a patient with an interleukin-1 receptor-associated kinase-4 (IRAK-4) mutation (PT) were treated with either lipopolysaccharide (LPS; 100 ng/mL) or formyl-methionyl-leucyl-phenylalanine (fMLF; 0.1 μM) for 30 minutes at 37°C. The cells were washed and stained with C10 (an antibody that demonstrates neutrophil heterogeneity), CD18, CD11b (antibodies to β2 integrins), CD66b (a specific granule marker), CD45 (the common leukocyte antigen), and L-selectin. The green lines represent the isotype control, blue lines represent control neutrophils, and purple lines represent stimulated cells. Differences between control and stimulated cells have been shaded. (From Kuhns DB, Long Priel DA, Gallin JI. Endotoxin and IL-1 hyporesponsiveness in a patient with recurrent bacterial infections. J Immunol 1997;158:3959, with permission of the American Association of Immunologists, Inc.)

supernatant fluid and the cell pellet should be analyzed to determine the percentage of enzyme released. To differentiate degranulation from cell lysis, release of the cytosolic enzyme lactate dehydrogenase should be monitored simultaneously.

The release of azurophilic granules can be assessed by determining the levels of myeloperoxidase or elastase. CD63 is also found in the membrane of azurophilic granules and migrates to the neutrophil surface after stimulation with fMLF in the presence of cytochalasin b. The release of specific granules can be assessed by determination of lactoferrin levels by using an enzyme-linked immunoassay. The carcinoembryonic antigen CD66b is found on the neutrophil surface and the specific granules, and its expression on the surface of the neutrophils is increased after stimulation with fMLF or LPS. The secretory granules usually contain proteins that are translocated into the membrane from cytosol during degranulation. Detection of the constituents of secretory granules can be assessed by flow cytometric analysis of the change in expression of surface proteins, such as adhesion molecules, and cytochrome b_{558} of the NADPH oxidase.

REACTIVE OXYGEN SPECIES GENERATION

Clinical Indications and Implications

The release of ROS, such as $O_2^{\cdot}$ and H_2O_2, is an important component of the bactericidal machinery of a neutrophil. Neutrophils isolated from patients with CGD have a defect in the NADPH oxidase and are unable to generate ROS, resulting in an O_2-dependent bactericidal defect. The production of ROS has become an important tool to perform risk assessment in patients with CGD. Patients with the lowest ROS generation ($<1\%$ of normal generation) have lower survival than patients with higher ROS generation ($3-10\%$ of normal). Moreover, survival in CGD is a continuous function of ROS production, suggesting that therapeutic interventions that result in an increase in ROS generation should incur a survival benefit to patients with CGD.[27]

Key Concepts
Reactive Oxygen Species in Chronic Granulomatous Disease

- Neutrophil reactive oxygen species (ROS) production, the primary determinate in diagnosis of patients with CGD, ranges from 0.1% to 27% of that observed in normal subjects.
- In addition, survival in chronic granulomatous disease (CGD) is strongly associated with residual ROS production as a continuous variable and is independent of the specific protein defect.
- ROS production is an important, early indicator of overall risk in CGD.
- In addition, small increases (as little as 3–5% of normal) in residual neutrophil ROS production may confer a survival benefit.
- Careful monitoring with detection of even small increases in ROS may be an important indicator of clinical efficacy during therapeutic intervention.

Principles and Interpretation of Laboratory Assessments

The nitroblue tetrazolium (NBT) test is a qualitative assay of ROS production. Either whole blood or isolated neutrophils are mixed with NBT in a chamber slide and stimulated with PMA for 15–30 minutes at 37°C. The neutrophils are allowed to settle on the slide. The slide is air-dried, counterstained with 0.1% safranin, and examined under a microscope. The NBT test yields a visual record of the reduction of the NBT dye to the insoluble, blue-black deposits of formazan. Normal neutrophils, but not neutrophils from patients with CGD, reduce the yellow dye to black-brown-blue aggregates in the cells. Because of the random inactivation of the X chromosome, X-linked carriers of CGD exhibit both NBT^+ and NBT^- neutrophils. The percentage of NBT^+ neutrophils in X-linked carriers of CGD ranges from 5 to 95%. The drawback of the NBT test is the need for manual counting to obtain an accurate reflection of the percentage of positive cells. An alternative to the NBT test is a flow cytometric assay using the dye dihydrorhodamine–123 (DHR-123).[28] Neutrophils are loaded with the nonfluorescent dye and then stimulated with PMA for 15 minutes at 37°C. The H_2O_2 produced oxidizes the dye and results in increased fluorescence, which is detectable with a flow cytometer. The assay is dependent on endogenous myeloperoxidase in the primary granules. Catalase is added to prevent cell-to-cell diffusion of H_2O_2. Since dye is localized to the cytoplasm and catalase is present in the extracellular fluid, the DHR-123 assay detects the intracellular production of ROS. As shown in Fig. 4.5, stimulation of normal neutrophils (Fig. 4.5A) with PMA results in a two-log shift in the fluorescence intensity. Neutrophils from an X-linked carrier of CGD (see Fig. 4.5B) exhibit mosaicism with a negatively stained (abnormal) population and a brightly stained positive population. Neutrophils from a patient with X-linked CGD that lack gp91^{phox} (Fig. 4.5C) express little increase in fluorescence while neutrophils from a patient with a deficiency in p47^{phox} (Fig. 4.5D) exhibit a slight increase in fluorescence. The major advantages of the DHR-123 assay are the sensitivity, the signal-to-noise ratio, and the ease of counting a large number of cells. Moreover, it has been shown that the DHR-123 assay yields reliable results on ethylenediaminetetraacetic acid (EDTA) or heparin-treated blood samples that have been stored overnight. In general, more than 90% of the neutrophils from the control blood samples will exhibit increased DHR-123 fluorescence. For this same reason, however, overnight samples should not be used to rule out X-linked heterozygosity, since a highly lyonized CGD carrier (>90%) could yield similar results.

The production of $O_2^{\cdot}$ can be detected using the reduction of cytochrome c. Because $O_2^{\cdot}$ causes a one-to-one stoichiometric reduction of ferricytochrome c to ferrocytochrome c, the resultant increase in the absorption spectrum at 550 nM can be used to

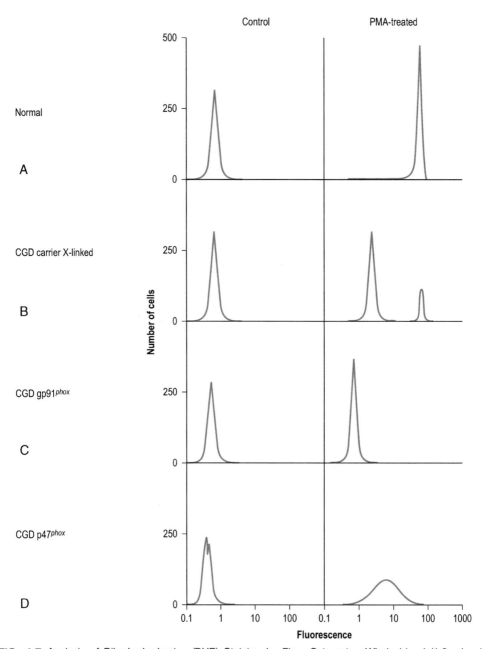

FIG. 4.5 Analysis of Dihydrorhodamine (DHR) Staining by Flow Cytometry. Whole blood (1.2 mL with ethylenediaminetetraacetic acid [EDTA] as anticoagulant) collected from a normal subject (A), an X-linked chronic granulomatous disease (CGD) carrier (B), a gp91^{phox} CGD patient (C), and a p47^{phox} CGD patient (D) was lysed by using an ammonium chloride-potassium bicarbonate solution. The remaining leukocytes were resuspended in HBSS and incubated with DHR-123 (100 μM) and catalase (50 μg/mL) for 5 minutes at 37°C. The cells were then incubated an additional 15 minutes at 37°C with either buffer (control) or phorbol myristate acetate (PMA; 400 ng/mL). The cells were immediately analyzed by flow cytometric analysis. Neutrophils were gated using forward light scattering and right-angle light scattering. The analyses presented represent 5000 events within the gated area.

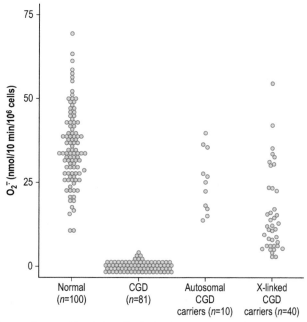

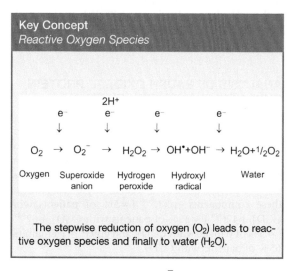

FIG. 4.6 Generation of Superoxide Anion Radicals From Normal Subjects, Patients With Chronic Granulomatous Disease (CGD), and Carriers of CGD. Neutrophils (1×10^6/mL in Hank's balanced salt solution [HBSS]) were incubated in the presence of 100 μM cytochrome c with phorbol myristate acetate (PMA; 100 ng/mL) for 10 minutes at 37°C. The reaction was terminated by centrifugation at 4°C. Reduction of cytochrome c was monitored at an analytical wavelength of 549.5 nm and a micromolar extinction coefficient of 0.0211. An identical tube containing superoxide dismutase (100 μg/mL) served as a blank.

quantitate the production of $O_2^{\cdot-}$. Superoxide dismutase is added to an identical tube to control for the nonspecific reduction of cytochrome c. However, since cytochrome is not permeable to the cells, the detection of $O_2^{\cdot}$ is limited to that released into the extracellular milieu. Neutrophils isolated from normal volunteers produce 0.42 ± 0.67 nmol/10^6 neutrophils/10 min under resting conditions; treatment with PMA results in 35.92 ± 11.92 nmol/10^6 neutrophils/10 min (Fig. 4.6). An estimate of normal $O_2^{\cdot}$ production over 60 minutes can be obtained by reducing the number of neutrophils in the assay to 2×10^5. Neutrophils isolated from patients with CGD produce little, if any, $O_2^{\cdot}$ in response to PMA in 10 minutes (Fig. 4.6). However, some patients with autosomal forms of CGD have low, but detectable, $O_2^{\cdot}$ production in 60 minutes. Neutrophils isolated from X-linked heterozygous carriers of CGD can yield a full spectrum of $O_2^{\cdot}$ production, whereas neutrophils from autosomal recessive carriers of CGD generally yield a normal response (Fig. 4.6). Although the detection of $O_2^{\cdot}$ by reduction of cytochrome c is useful in the diagnosis of patients with CGD, it cannot be used in the diagnosis of carriers because of the wide spectrum of

responses that result from the degree of X chromosome lyonization.

Key Concept
Reactive Oxygen Species

$$O_2 \rightarrow O_2^{-} \rightarrow H_2O_2 \rightarrow OH^{\cdot}+OH^{-} \rightarrow H_2O+\tfrac{1}{2}O_2$$

| Oxygen | Superoxide anion | Hydrogen peroxide | Hydroxyl radical | Water |

The stepwise reduction of oxygen (O_2) leads to reactive oxygen species and finally to water (H_2O).

Studies have shown that $O_2^{\cdot}$ determinations sufficiently reliable to diagnose CGD can be obtained from neutrophils isolated from heparinized whole blood that has been stored overnight. Hence, analyses can be performed on blood samples shipped by overnight express. A normal control blood sample should accompany the sample to ensure adequate shipment handling. By 48 hours of storage, however, there are marked reductions in the PMA response, and the data are no longer valid.

An alternative assay to measure ROS production is luminol-enhanced chemiluminescence. This versatile assay, in addition to its quick and easy setup, offers the capability to test several different subjects and stimuli on the same plate using reduced numbers of cells while providing high sensitivity. The luminescence readings are taken every 1–5 min for up to 2 hours, and data are expressed as relative light units (RLUs). Different stimuli exhibit different kinetics (*e.g.*, fMLF induces a rapid respiratory burst that decays quickly, whereas PMA [20–100 ng/mL] induces a peak of luminescence within 5–15 minutes that slowly decays by 2 hours). Results from normal subjects and patients can be assessed simultaneously and monitored kinetically or using the area under the curve (AUC). Luminol-enhanced chemiluminescence is a measure of both intracellular and extracellular ROS production, although it may not detect them with equivalent efficiency. Addition of superoxide dismutase significantly reduces both peak height and AUC after stimulation with PMA, suggesting that at least a portion of the response can be attributed to $O_2^{\cdot-}$. Typically, patients with CGD who are deficient in gp91^{phox} have little to no detectable luminescence in this assay; however, as observed with the ferricytochrome c assay, patients with CGD who are deficient in p47^{phox} have detectable luminescence that becomes most evident at later readings (40–80 minutes) (Fig. 4.7).

ANALYSIS OF NADPH OXIDASE PROTEIN SUBUNITS BY WESTERN BLOTTING
Clinical Indications and Implications
The NADPH oxidase consists of two membrane components (p22^{phox} and gp91^{phox}), three cytosolic components (p47^{phox}, p67^{phox}, and p40^{phox}), and several guanosine triphosphate (GTP)–binding proteins. CGD is characterized by defects in any one of four of these components—p22^{phox} ($\approx 5\%$ of patients with CGD), p47^{phox} ($\approx 25\%$ of patients with CGD), p67^{phox} ($\approx 5\%$ of patients with CGD), and gp91^{phox} (remaining 65% of patients with CGD).

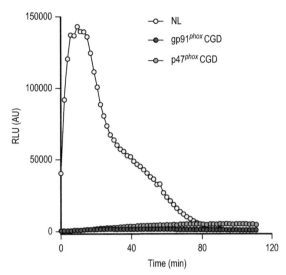

FIG. 4.7 Neutrophil Luminol–Enhanced Chemiluminescence. Neutrophils (1 x 10^5/200 μL) were preloaded with luminol (100 μM) for 10 min at 37°C. At t = 0, either buffer or phorbol myristate acetate (PMA; 100 ng/mL) was added and luminescence was monitored for 2 hours, with readings recorded every 2 minutes. Note that at later readings, neutrophils from a patient with p47^{phox} deficiency had increased luminescence compared with neutrophils from a patient with chronic granulomatous disease (CGD) gp91^{phox} deficiency.

Principles and Interpretation of Laboratory Assessments
The severity of CGD can be related to the specific protein defect. Determination of the specific protein defect in CGD by Western blot analysis also provides direction for determination of the specific genetic defect and enables appropriate genetic counseling for the extended family. A validated normal control is included on each gel for band identification and intensity comparisons. In addition, a control sample from a patient with a known mutation in gp91^{phox} CGD is included on each blot to ensure adequate development of p22^{phox}. Typical phox protein band patterns are presented in Fig. 4.8. Patients with CGD who have mutations in p47^{phox} are Western blot negative. Patients with CGD who have mutations in p67^{phox} are generally Western blot negative; however, we have analyzed one patient with a missense mutation in p67^{phox} who was Western blot positive. Because p22^{phox} and gp91^{phox}

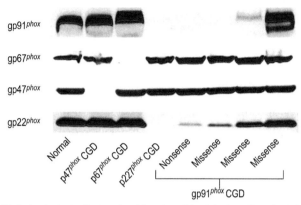

FIG. 4.8 Western Blot Analysis to Determine Nicotinamide Adenine Dinucleotide Phosphate (NADPH) Oxidase Protein Defect. Frozen, diisopropylflurophosphate (DFP)–treated neutrophil pellets (5×10^6 cells) were resuspended in polyacrylamide gel electrophoresis (PAGE) sample buffer and sonicated to break up the DNA. One million cell equivalents were loaded into each lane (10% PAGE gels for p47^{phox} and p67^{phox}, 4–12% gradient PAGE gels for p22^{phox} and gp91^{phox}). A validated normal control was run on each gel for quality control. The gels were transferred to nitrocellulose, blocked with 5% powdered milk, and incubated overnight with specific antibodies to the phox proteins. The blots were washed, incubated with peroxidase-labeled secondary antibody, and developed with a color reagent. The blots were scanned for permanent storage, and a composite figure was created by using the relevant bands from each blot. The lanes are identified by the specific protein defect and, for gp91^{phox}, the type of mutation. CGD, chronic granulomatous disease.

exist as a membrane complex, patients with a defect in p22^{phox} are generally Western blot negative for both p22^{phox} and gp91^{phox}. In contrast, defects in gp91^{phox} yield more variable results. In general, patients with nonsense defects in gp91^{phox} exhibit low but detectable levels of p22^{phox}. Patients with missense mutations in gp91^{phox} that yield detectable gp91^{phox} protein exhibit proportionately higher levels of p22^{phox}. Neutrophils isolated from overnight samples can be used to diagnose p47^{phox} deficiency because of the stability of the protein. However, detection of other phox protein defects in overnight samples can be more problematic because of proteolysis of p67^{phox} and the gp91^{phox}-p22^{phox} complex.

CONCLUSIONS

On the Horizon

There is growing evidence that neutrophils may be derived from organs other than bone marrow, such as the lung, liver, and, particularly, spleen. Recently, it has been suggested that the spleen may serve as a reserve site for "emergency myelopoiesis" during infection. Other studies suggest that c-kit$^+$ myeloid precursors from blood migrate to a site of cutaneous infection, where they proliferate and form mature polymorphonuclear neutrophils

(PMNs). These findings are based on murine studies and raise the following questions:

- Are these extramedullary neutrophils found in humans?
- Are there specific biomarkers that distinguish them from their bone marrow–derived circulating counterparts?
- Do they have functionality that is different from circulating neutrophils?

Our understanding of neutrophil biology is undergoing significant changes. Long-standing axioms are being challenged. Chakravarti et al. suggested that treatment of neutrophils with a cocktail of cytokines can reprogram a phenotypically distinct subset of neutrophils with increased survival and altered function.[29] Rodriguez et al. have shown that patients with renal cancer have a subset of lighter density neutrophils that colocalize with mononuclear cells atop the density cushion and appear to be phenotypically "activated"[30]; moreover, these lighter-density neutrophils are capable of suppressing T-cell proliferation through a mechanism dependent on arginase-1 stored in the gelatinase granules, a novel function of neutrophils.

Much of our current understanding of neutrophil biology has developed from the study of genetic immunodeficiencies. Whether there are immunodeficiencies that result from defects in these recently discovered pathways has yet to be determined.

ACKNOWLEDGMENT

This project has been funded in whole or in part with federal funds from the National Cancer Institute, National Institutes of Health, under Contract HHSN261200800001E. The content of this publication does not necessarily reflect the views or policies of the Department of Health and Human Services, nor does mention of trade names, commercial products, or organizations imply endorsement by the US Government.

REFERENCES

1. Jhunjhunwala S, Alvarez D, Aresta-DaSilva S, et al. Splenic progenitors aid in maintaining high neutrophil numbers at sites of sterile chronic inflammation. *J Leukocyte Biol.* 2016;100:253–260.
2. Bainton DF. The cells of inflammation: a general view. In: Weissman G, ed. *The Cell Biology of Inflammation.* 2nd ed. New York: Elsevier/North-Holland; 1980.
3. Pillay JP, den Braber I, Vrisekoop N, et al. *In vivo* labeling with ^2H_2O reveals a human neutrophil lifespan of 5.4 days. *Blood.* 2010;116(4):625–627.
4. Borregaard N, Cowland JB. Granules of the human neutrophilic polymorphonuclear leukocyte. *Blood.* 1997;89:3503–3521.
5. Volpp BD, Nauseef WM, Clark RA. Two cytosolic neutrophil oxidase components absent in autosomal chronic granulomatous disease. *Science.* 1988;242:1295–1297.
6. Matute JD, Arias AA, Wright NAM, et al. A new genetic subgroup of chronic granulomatous disease with autosomal recessive mutations in p40^{phox} and selective defects in neutrophil NADPH oxidase activity. *Blood.* 2009;114:3309–3315.
7. Parkos CA, Dinauer MC, Walker LE, et al. Primary structure and unique expression of the 22-kilodalton light chain of human neutrophil cytochrome b. *Proc Natl Acad Sci USA.* 1988;85:3319–3323.
8. Segal AW, Cross AR, Garcia RC, et al. Absence of cytochrome b-$_{245}$ in chronic granulomatous disease—a multicenter European evaluation of its incidence and relevance. *N Engl J Med.* 1983;308:245–251.
9. Thomas DC. The phagocyte respiratory burst: historical perspectives and recent advances. *Immunol Lett.* 2017;192:88–96.
10. Brinkmann V, Reichard U, Goosmann C, et al. Neutrophil extracellular traps kill bacteria. *Science.* 2004;303:1532–1535.
11. Lood C, Blanco LP, Purmalek MM, et al. Neutrophil extracellular traps enriched in oxidized mitochondrial DNA are interferogenic and contribute to lupus-like disease. *Nat Med.* 2016;27:146–153.
12. Lanini LL, Prader S, Siler U, et al. Modern management of phagocyte defects. *Pediatr Allergy Immunol.* 2017;28:124–134.
13. Kuijpers TW, Tool ATJ, van der Schoot CE, et al. Membrane surface antigen expression on neutrophils: a reappraisal of the use of surface markers for neutrophil activation. *Blood.* 1991;78:1105–1111.
14. Böyum A. Isolation of mononuclear cells and granulocytes from human blood. Isolation of monuclear cells by one centrifugation, and of granulocytes by combining centrifugation and sedimentation at 1 g. *Scand J Clin Invest Suppl.* 1968;97:77–89.
15. Haslett C, Guthrie LA, Kopaniak MM, et al. Modulation of multiple neutrophil functions by preparative methods or trace concentrations of bacterial lipopolysaccharide. *Am J Pathol.* 1985;119:101–110.
16. Kaplow LS. Simplified myeloperoxidase stain using benzidine dihydrochloride. *Blood.* 1965;26:215–219.
17. Introne W, Boissy REB, Gahl WA. Clinical, molecular, and cell biological aspects of Chediak–Higashi syndrome. *Mol Genet Metab.* 1999;68:283–303.
18. Strauss RG, Bove KE, Jones JF, et al. An anomaly of neutrophil morphology with impaired function. *NEJM.* 1974;290:478–484.
19. Nauseef WM. Diagnostic assays for myeloperoxidase deficiency. In: Quinn MT, DeLeo FR, Bokoch GM, eds. *Neutrophil Methods and Protocols: Methods in Molecular Biology.* Totowa, NJ: Humana Press; 2007:525–530.
20. Parmley RT, Gilbert CS, Boxer LA. Abnormal peroxidase-positive granules in "specific granule" deficiency. *Blood.* 1989;73:838–844.
21. Buescher ES, Gaither T, Nath J, et al. Abnormal adherence-related functions of neutrophils, monocytes, and Epstein-Barr virus-transformed B cells in a patient with C3bi receptor deficiency. *Blood.* 1985;65:1382–1390.
22. Anderson DC, Schmalstieg FC, Finegold MJ, et al. The severe and moderate phenotypes of heritable Mac-1, LFA-1 deficiency: their quantitative definition and relation to leukocyte dysfunction and clinical features. *J Infect Dis.* 1985;152:668–689.
23. Etzioni A, Frydman M, Pollack S, et al. Recurrent severe infections caused by a novel leukocyte adhesion deficiency. *N Engl J Med.* 1992;327:1789–1792.
24. Frevert CW, Wong VA, Goodman RB, et al. Rapid fluorescence-based measurement of neutrophil migration *in vitro. J Immunol Methods.* 1998;213:41–52.
25. Anderson DC, Springer TA. Leukocyte adhesion deficiency: an inherited defect in the Mac-1, LFA-1, and p150,95 glycoproteins. *Annu Rev Med.* 1987;38:175–194.

26. Kuhns DB, Long Priel DA, Gallin JI. Endotoxin and IL-1 hyporesponsiveness in a patient with recurrent bacterial infections. *J Immunol.* 1997;158:3959—3964.

27. Kuhns DB, Alvord WG, Heller T, et al. Residual NADPH oxidase and survival in chronic granulomatous disease. *N Engl J Med.* 2010;363:2600—2610.

28. Emmendörffer A, Hecht M, Lohmann-Matthes M-L, et al. A fast and easy method to determine the production of reactive oxygen intermediates by human and murine phagocytes using dihydrorhodamine 123. *J Immunol Methods.* 1990;131:269—275.

29. Chakravarti A, Rusu D, Flamand N, et al. Reprogramming of a subpopulation of human blood neutrophils by prolonged exposure to cytokines. *Lab Investig.* 2009;89:1084—1099.

30. Rodriguez PC, Ernstoff MS, Hernandez C, et al. Arginase I-producing myeloid-derived suppressor cells in renal cell carcinoma are a subpopulation of activated granulocytes. *Cancer Res.* 2009;15:1553—1560.

CHAPTER 5

Investigation of Allergic Diseases In Vitro

ROBERT G. HAMILTON

Human allergic disease comprises a spectrum of immunoglobulin E (IgE)—mediated immediate-type hypersensitivity reactions that manifest as reactions in skin (urticaria, dermatitis), the respiratory tract (asthma, rhinitis, or sinusitis), eyes (conjunctivitis), the gastrointestinal (GI) tract (abdominal pain, bloating, vomiting, diarrhea), and, in their most extreme condition, systemic anaphylaxis. These reactions are precipitated by exposure of a genetically predisposed and sensitized (IgE antibody-positive) individual to a variety of environmental substances that are ubiquitous and usually well tolerated by most healthy individuals. This chapter reviews the principles and performance characteristics of *in vitro* analytical methods used in the diagnosis and management of individuals with allergic disease.

BIOLOGICAL PROPERTIES OF IgE

In 1921, Prausnitz and Küstner (PK)[1] reported that an intradermal (ID) injection of serum from an allergic individual into the skin of an unsensitized (nonallergic) individual, followed 24 hours later by injection of specific antigen into the same skin site, induced local itching and swelling surrounded by a zone of erythema. This passively transferred allergic reaction, or *PK reaction*, reached a maximum within 10 minutes, persisted for about 20 minutes, and gradually disappeared. The antibody mediating this reaction was shown to be thermolabile, losing its sensitizing activity after heating serum at 56°C for several hours. In 1967, this antibody was identified as a fifth human immunoglobulin isotype and designated as IgE.[2—4]

Total serum IgE concentrations are the lowest of the five human immunoglobulin isotypes (0—0.0001 g/L; 0.004% of the total adult serum immunoglobulin).[5] Approximately 50% of IgE is localized in the extravascular space. Its short biological half-life of 1—5 days in peripheral blood is primarily the result of a relatively high fractional catabolic rate (71% of the intravascular pool catabolized/day). IgE does not pass the placenta or activate the classical complement pathway. Its reaginic (mast-cell sensitizing) activity is dependent on its ability to bind to the α chain of the high-affinity IgE Fc-ε receptor (α-FcεRI) that resides on the membrane surface of basophils and mast cells. The interaction between IgE Fc and the α-FcεRI is blocked by the therapeutic subcutaneous administration of anti-IgE therapeutics, such as omalizumab (a humanized IgG1-κ anti-IgE Fc), as discussed below.

CLINICAL IMPORTANCE OF TOTAL SERUM IgE

The concentration of IgE in the serum is highly age dependent.[5] Cord serum IgE concentrations are low, usually <2 kU/L (<4.88 μg/L; 1 kU = 2.44 μg and 1 IU = 2.44 ng). Serum IgE levels progressively increase in healthy children up to the age of 10—15 years and gradually decline in an age-dependent manner from the second to the eighth decades of life. Infants with atopia have an earlier and steeper rise in serum IgE levels during their early years compared with age-matched controls without atopia.[6]

Clinically, a patient's total serum IgE level should be evaluated against reference intervals established with sera from an age-stratified, healthy skin test-negative (nonatopic) population.[6] Many clinical laboratories define a total serum IgE >100 kU/L (240 ng/mL) as a general demarcation into the atopic region.[7] After the age of 14 years, serum IgE levels >333 kU/l (>800 μg/L) are abnormally elevated and strongly associated with atopic disorders, such as allergic rhinitis, extrinsic or allergic asthma, and atopic dermatitis. Extreme elevations in serum IgE are common in parasitic infections and are necessary for the diagnosis of the hyper-IgE (Job's) syndrome. Low total IgE

Core Laboratory Technologies in Clinical Immunology. https://doi.org/10.1016/B978-0-323-66149-2.00005-0

levels <25 kU/L in individuals with asthma suggest that IgE-mediated mechanisms play an insignificant role in the pathogenesis of their condition. Low total serum IgE levels thus support the diagnosis of nonallergic (intrinsic) asthma and help exclude allergic broncho-pulmonary aspergillosis. There is extensive overlap between IgE levels in atopic and nonatopic populations,[6−9] which means that an elevated serum IgE can be useful in confirming the clinical diagnosis of allergic respiratory or skin diseases, but a low or normal value does not eliminate the possibility of an IgE-mediated mechanism. For instance, a group of adults with allergic asthma had a mean serum IgE level of 1589 ng/mL (range 55−12 750 ng/mL). In contrast, approximately 90% of patients with atopic dermatitis had elevated total serum IgE levels (mean 978 kU/L; range 1.3−65,208 kU/L). Parasitic infections, selected immunodeficiency states, cancer (Hodgkin disease, bronchial carcinoma), rheumatoid arthritis, liver disease, and atopic dermatitis (eczema) are other disease states that have been associated with a dysregulation of total serum IgE levels. The total serum IgE must therefore be interpreted within the relevant clinical context for each patient.

Because of the overlap between individuals with atopia and those without, total serum IgE measurements have been largely replaced in the routine diagnosis of allergic disease by the quantification of allergen-specific IgE antibody. However, quantification of total serum IgE has remained important for computing the therapeutic dose of anti-IgE. Omalizumab is a recombinant, humanized IgG1-κ monoclonal antihuman IgE Fc drug that specifically binds to the region on the ε heavy chain that interacts with α-FcεR1.[10,11] It is used to treat moderate to severe persistent allergic asthma and chronic idiopathic urticaria by blocking IgE binding to the α-FcεR1. The binding of omalizumab to IgE *in vivo* reduces both the number of free IgE molecules able to interact with the α-FcεR1 and the number of α-FcεR1 receptors on the surface of effector cells. The consequence is a reduction in mediator release and allergy symptoms following allergen exposure.[10,11]

CLINICAL IMPORTANCE OF ALLERGEN-SPECIFIC IgE

In contrast to total serum IgE, the presence of allergen-specific IgE antibody on the surface of circulating basophils or skin mast cells or in the serum is highly predictive of an individual's propensity to exhibit an allergic response following reexposure to that allergen.

Before its identification as a novel immunoglobulin, IgE was only detectable with *in vivo* bioassays (skin test, bronchial or nasal provocation tests). Purification of IgE myeloma protein and the subsequent production of antisera specific for IgE led to the development of the first *in vitro* assay (radioallergosorbent test [RAST]) for the detection of allergen-specific IgE antibody in serum.[4,12,13] Since then, nonisotopic autoanalyzer variants based on the original noncompetitive cellulose paper disc solid-phase RAST design have been widely used in clinical immunology laboratories throughout the world.[13,14] These assays, discussed below, involve an immobilized allergen containing reagent that binds allergen-specific antibody from human serum and an enzyme conjugated anti-IgE that detects bound IgE antibody.

Historical studies have compared the diagnostic performance (sensitivity and specificity) of *in vivo* and the *in vitro* assays in the diagnosis of human allergic disease. These intermethod comparisons have shown that the presence of IgE antibody as measured by serological immunoassay methods usually agrees well with the presence of IgE detected in leukocyte and mast-cell histamine release assays, and provocation tests, such as the skin test, food challenge, and inhalation provocation test.[15,16] However, these early studies emphasize that the presence of IgE antibody as detected either *in vivo* or *in vitro* is at best a confirmatory measurement for sensitization.[17] IgE antibody is necessary but not sufficient for induction of an allergic symptom. It is considered an important risk factor in the diagnosis of allergic disease that supports a patient's medical, family, and environmental histories of a temporal association between allergic symptoms and allergen exposure. The clinical importance of differences in diagnostic sensitivity between skin test and serological detection of IgE antibody may be less important for patients with allergies to inhaled (pollen, dust mite, and epidermal) allergens than in those facing life-threatening anaphylactic reactions caused by *Hymenoptera* stings and certain drugs. In these latter cases, skin tests are preferable to *in vitro* immunoassay analyses for the detection of allergen-specific IgE antibodies.[16,18] Immunoassays of IgE antibody in serum can, however, be helpful in cases where the patient has taken antihistamines, β-receptor stimulants, or high-dose steroids, which can reduce the *in vivo* provocation test's measured response in children, pregnant women, and older patients, in whom skin testing may not be well tolerated and when dealing with allergens (*e.g.*, foods, molds) where commercial extracts can be highly variable or labile.[13,16]

DIAGNOSTIC METHODS

A combination of *in vivo* provocation and *in vitro* laboratory tests may be used to confirm sensitization and provide support for the clinical diagnosis of allergic disease. The actual tests selected depend on the nature of the disease process (*e.g.*, allergic asthma, urticaria/angioedema, rhinitis/sinusitis, or anaphylaxis) and the suspected allergen triggers (*e.g.*, aeroallergens, venoms, drugs, foods) under investigation. In making a decision about which diagnostic test to perform, clinicians start by searching for information on the diagnostic sensitivity and specificity of each confirmatory test. The true *diagnostic sensitivity* or ability of each test to detect IgE antibody in the presence of allergic disease and *diagnostic specificity* or ability of the test to not detect IgE antibody in health (absence of allergic disease) are difficult to determine definitively. Not only are there a myriad of assay methods, diverse techniques (*e.g.*, skin testing), reagents (extracts and molecules) and grading, interpolation, and interpretation methods, but most importantly, there is a general absence of gold standard methods for defining the presence of allergic disease. For this reason, results of the confirmatory tests need to be viewed as additional risk factors and tests for sensitization, rather than definitive indicators of disease.[17] In the end, the choice of the confirmatory test is a matter of clinical judgment.

INITIAL CLINICAL LABORATORY TESTS

Following the collection of a medical history and performance of a physical examination, the patient who is suspected of having allergic disease may undergo several preliminary blood tests. A complete blood count (CBC), and/or a total blood eosinophil count, if performed, should be obtained before any systemic corticosteroids or epinephrine is administered. A normal whole blood eosinophil level ranges from 0 to 500 cells/mm^3. Children generally have higher normal levels (mean 240 cells/mm^3, 95% confidence interval, [CI] = 0−740 cells/mm^3), with peak levels occurring at 4−8 years of age. Most clinical laboratories consider a differential white blood cell (WBC) count with an eosinophil proportion >5−10% of the total WBC count to be abnormal. Blood, sputum, and nasal secretion eosinophilia are characteristic of asthma, whether or not IgE-mediated allergic processes are present. In a bronchitic sputum specimen, neutrophils predominate. A neutrophilic nasal discharge is characteristic of sinusitis. Other laboratory tests that may be ordered, as indicated, include pulmonary function tests and a chest X-ray or sinus computer tomography (CT) scan.

IN VIVO PROVOCATION TESTING

Both the skin test and nasal/bronchial/GI provocation tests are useful *in vivo* diagnostic tools for the confirmation of immediate-type hypersensitivity reactions associated with allergic disease. They can also allow the identification of offending allergens in an allergy patient's workup for avoidance, or management with pharmacotherapy, immunotherapy, or anti-IgE therapy. Details of skin testing are outside the scope of this chapter but are available elsewhere.[19]

Key Concepts
Immunoglobulin E (IgE) (Reaginic) Antibody Detection

- Allergen-specific IgE can be detected by skin test using a puncture or intradermal administration of allergen or in the serum by laboratory-based immunoassays.
- In general, the intradermal (ID) skin test is more analytically sensitive than a puncture skin test, which is roughly comparable to the best *in vitro* methods for IgE antibody detection in serum.
- ID skin tests are the diagnostic procedure of choice in the workup of patients with suspected *Hymenoptera* venom and drug allergy, while both *in vitro* and *in vivo* assay methods are complementary for evaluating aeroallergen-related disease.
- Serological analyses of IgE antibody—specific for food allergens are often favored over extract-based skin test analyses in part because of more enhanced reagent quality control; however, the double-blind placebo-controlled food challenge (DBPCFC) remains the gold standard for definitive diagnosis of food allergies.
- IgE antibody to allergenic molecules (components) can in some cases (*e.g.*, peanut, hazelnut) provide clarity in terms of the specificity of the patient's sensitization profile (genuine vs. cross-reactivity) and relative risk for mild versus serious systemic reactions.

IN VITRO TESTING

Clinical immunology laboratories worldwide offer serological tests that are useful in the diagnosis and management of human allergic disease. Analytes commonly measured in these laboratories include the total serum IgE, IgE antibodies to hundreds of allergen specificities, *Hymenoptera* venom-specific IgG, the IgE antivenom-inhibition test, and mast-cell tryptase. IgG antibody measurements to allergens other than *Hymenoptera* venom have not been shown to be clinically useful.[20] Basophil mediator and activation tests, although rarely offered as clinical tests because of the requirement for fresh blood, are useful investigational methods that are also reviewed in this section.

Total Serum IgE

Of the diagnostic allergy tests that are performed in the clinical immunology laboratory, total serum IgE is currently the only diagnostic allergy analyte regulated under the US Clinical Laboratory Improvement Amendment of 1988 (CLIA-88). Current commercial assays to measure the total level of IgE in serum employ nonisotopic labels, such as enzymes (horseradish peroxidase, alkaline phosphatase, β-galactosidase) or fluorophores, and have been cleared by the US Food and Drug Administration (FDA). The minimum detectable concentration of the commercial total serum IgE assays is between 0.5 and 1 μg/L. The intermethod agreement of the different commercial IgE assays is excellent (*e.g.*, intermethod coefficients of variation [CVs] typically <15%).[13,21] Nonatopic age-adjusted reference intervals for total serum IgE must be used for normative interpretation.[5]

Total IgE Measurements After Therapeutic Anti-IgE Administration

Omalizumab (anti-IgE) is currently used as a fourth therapeutic modality to supplement avoidance, pharmacotherapy, and immunotherapy in the management of persistent asthma and urticaria, and off-label for other IgE-mediated states (*e.g.*, allergic bronchopulmonary aspergillosis, pretreatment of food allergy patients receiving immunotherapy). Since its conception,[22] clinicians have desired to quantify the level of total and "free" (uncomplexed) IgE in anti-IgE-treated patients as a rationale for treatment failures or to justify modification of a patient's dosing regimen to maximize treatment success. A systematic evaluation of the impact of therapeutic anti-IgE on the performance of clinically used total IgE assays showed variable interference that resulted in a 1.9–51.9% reduction in accuracy, depending on the assay.[23] Accurate quantitation of the level of uncomplexed or "free" IgE in the serum of treated patients has been more technically difficult. The performance of the existing free IgE assays has been heavily criticized,[24] leading some investigators to a conclusion that there may be no simple and analytically accurate clinical method for quantifying the level of free IgE in the serum of patients who have received omalizumab. This, however, may change with a new anti-IgE therapeutic that has been engineered so it is removed from circulation once it complexes IgE.[25]

Allergen-Specific IgE

Laboratories in the United States that perform clinical diagnostic allergy testing must be federally licensed, use a United States FDA-cleared assay method, and perform successfully in an external diagnostic allergy proficiency survey (*e.g.*, College of American Pathologists [CAP] SE Survey).[13,21] These assays, which have been through rigorous validation, have achieved unsurpassed intraassay precision, interassay reproducibility, and a high degree of quantification.[13] Their basic design can be traced to the first IgE antibody assay, the RAST, reported by Wide et al. in 1967.[12]

Allergen

The most highly variable component of the IgE antibody assay is the allergen-containing reagent. Allergens are mixtures of molecules, typically proteins, glycoproteins, lipoproteins, or protein-conjugate chemicals or drugs that have been solubilized from a defined (usually biological) source, a portion of which can elicit an IgE antibody response in exposed and genetically predisposed individuals. They possess common properties of stability to processing (*e.g.*, heat) and digestion because of multiple cysteine linkages. They tend to be abundant in nature, form aggregates or polymers, commonly interact with lipid structures, and serve to defend their biological source. Cross-tabulation of the protein family (PFAM) database (n = 16 230 protein families) with the Structural Database of Allergenic Proteins (SDAP) identified 130 PFAMs in the Allergenic Family database of allergenic proteins. Thus importantly, allergens comprise a small fraction of protein families with particular structures and biological functions.[26] The Clinical and Laboratory Standards Institute (CLSI) has an established international guidance document that defines the expected performance characteristics of allergenic materials used in immunological assays for human IgE antibodies.[13] It provides a compendium of the genus and species of all the allergen specificities of clinical interest, subdividing them into extract and component allergens and indicating whether they are well-documented or rare. They are categorized on the basis of their sources, into weed pollen, grass pollen, tree pollen, animal dander, mold, house dust mite fecal material, parasites, insect venoms, occupational allergens, foods, and drugs. Except for drugs, these extracts are complex heterogeneous mixtures that contain both nonallergenic and allergenic proteins. Some allergens share structural similarity or cross-reactive epitopes, and others possess unique IgE antibody-binding determinants. Among the different species of a genus, such as ragweed (*e.g.*, Canyon,

Desert, Giant, Short, Silver, Southern, Western), there is extensive allergenic cross-reactivity resulting from structural similarity. Extensive allergenic cross-reactivity has also been documented within other pollen groups, such as the grasses (June, Brome, Timothy, Perennial Rye, Fescue, Orchard, Red Top, Salt, Sweet Vernal, Velvet). In contrast, other grass pollens, such as those produced by Bermuda Grass, Johnson Grass, and cultivated corn, oat, and wheat, are minimally cross-reactive (allergenically distinct). Variations in the allergenic content of extracted source materials, the extraction process from the raw source material, allergen-reagent manufacturing methods, differential binding to various allergosorbent supports, instability during storage, heterogeneity of internal reference allergen standards, and differences in characterization procedures (antisera, assays) make the production of reproducible allergens for *in vitro* use a challenge.

Cross-reactivity has also been shown at the allergen component level. There are 10 principal allergen families that show structural similarity and extensive cross-reactivity (Table 5.1).[26,27] The most prominent is illustrated by the pathogenesis-related (PR)-10 family of allergens, also known as the *Bet v 1 homologues*. These are small (17-kDa) proteins in many plant species that transport steroids and exhibit low stability at high pH and in the presence of digestive enzymes. The first allergen in this family was identified from birch pollen (Bet v 1). Others with high amino acid sequence homology include Cor a 1-hazelnut, Mal d 1-apple, Pru p 1-peach, Gly m 4-soybean, Ara h 8-peanut, Aln g 1-alder, Act d 8-kiwi, Api g 1-celery, and Dau c 1-carrot. Other component based cross-reactivity groups include the profilins, nonspecific lipid transfer proteins, tropomyosins, serum albumins, polcalcins, lipocalins, parvalbumins, storage-binding proteins, and carbohydrate cross-reactive determinants (CCDs) (see Table 5.1). Each of these cross-reactive allergen families is extensively discussed in the *Handbook on Molecular Allergology*.[28]

Calibration

The second attribute that varies widely among commercially available IgE antibody assays is calibration algorithm and methodology. There exists no internationally recognized polyclonal human IgE antibody reference preparation. Thus all three autoanalyzers

---

TABLE 5.1
Principal Allergen Families and Their Associated Biological Functions

Family	Function	Diagnostic Utility and Clinical Features	Examples
Profilins	Actin-binding proteins involved in the dynamic turnover and restructuring of the actin cytoskeleton. Highly conserved, extremely cross-reactive, and ubiquitous proteins in pollen and plant foods	Positive skin test and immunoglobulin E (IgE) responses to (nonrelated) pollen species (often including grasses) and plant food extracts are indicative for IgE cross-reactivity to profilins. After proof of sensitization to one profilin pollen and plant food extracts are of no further use because of their subsequent lack of analytical specificity	Bet v 2 (birch); Phl p 12 (Timothy-grass); Hev b 8 (natural rubber latex); Mal d 4 (apple)
Serum albumins	Highly cross-reactive plasma protein carriers involved in transport of hormones, enzymes, hemin, and fatty acids. Also maintains oncotic pressure	Positive skin test and IgE responses to furred animals indicate IgE cross-reactivity to mammalian serum albumins. Proof of sensitizations to one serum albumin can explain clinical symptoms to rarely or uncooked meat ("cat-pork syndrome")	Fel d 2 (cat); Can f 3 (dog)

Continued

TABLE 5.1
Principal Allergen Families and Their Associated Biological Functions—cont'd

Family	Function	Diagnostic Utility and Clinical Features	Examples
Pathogenesis-related protein family 10 (PR-10), Bet v 1 homolog	Plant defense proteins; Bet v 1 is a quercetin-3-O-sophoroside-binding molecule (17 kDa); inflammation response proteins	Positive Bet v 1-specific IgE reflects sensitization to fagales tree pollen (*i.e.,* hazel, alder, birch, beech, oak). Thermo and digestion labile Bet v 1-homologs in fruits, legumes, and vegetables. Bet v 1-sensitized individuals can cause predominantly oropharyngeal symptoms after consumption of raw food items (*i.e.,* pip fruits, stone fruits, tree nuts, carrots, soy)	Bet v 1 (birch); Cor a 1 (hazelnut); Mal d 1 (apple); Gly m 4 (soy)
Polcalcin	Cross-reactive, ubiquitous, and calcium-binding proteins in pollen; involved in calcium regulation	Positive skin test and IgE responses to (nonrelated) pollen species are indicative for IgE cross-reactivity to polcalcins. After proof of sensitization to one, polcalcin pollen extracts are of no further use because of their subsequent lack of analytical specificity	Phl p 7 (Timothy-grass); Bet v 4 (birch); Amb a 10 (short ragweed)
Nonspecific lipid transfer proteins (nsLTP, PR-14)	Inflammation response proteins; responsible for shuttling phospholipids and other fatty acids between cell membranes	Primary food allergen after sensitization to peach lipid transfer protein (LTP) (possibly through the skin?); predominantly found in the Mediterranean subjects; variable degree of cross-reactivity between the thermally stable LTPs in fruits and vegetables causing frequently oropharyngeal and sometimes systemic symptoms (*i.e.,* exercise-induced)	Pru p 3 (peach); Ara h 9 (peanut); Cor a 8 (hazelnut)
Lipocalins	A highly heterogeneous group of extracellular proteins within various subfamilies involved in transport of small hydrophobic molecules, such as steroids, bilins, retinoids, and lipids	Positive skin test and IgE responses to more than one or many furred animals are indicative for IgE sensitization and subsequent serological cross-reactivity to lipocalins of a certain subfamily. As a consequence animal extracts are of no further use because of their subsequent lack of analytical specificity	Fel d 4, 7 (cat); Can f 1, 2, 4, 6 (dog)

TABLE 5.1
Principal Allergen Families and Their Associated Biological Functions—cont'd

Family	Function	Diagnostic Utility and Clinical Features	Examples
Parvalbumins	Calcium-binding proteins; localized in fast-contracting muscles and being involved in calcium signaling	Thermostable and digestion-stable major fish allergen with fairly high, but not complete cross-reactivity and high abundance in almost all fish species. Only limited sequence homology and no cross-reactivity between fish and shellfish Ca^{++}-binding proteins	Gad c 1 (cod); Cra c 4, 6 (shrimp)
Tropomyosins	Integral components of actin filament that play a role in regulating muscle contraction. Also regulate actin filament stability in nonmuscle cells	Thermostable and digestion-stable major shellfish allergen with broad cross-reactivity and high abundance in all shellfish species. IgE sensitization is associated with allergic reactions to various panels of shellfish species	Der p 10 (dust mite); Pen m 1 (shrimp)
Seed storage proteins	Heterodimeric, stable, and highly abundant proteins involved in nutrient storage: e.g., 2S albumins, 7/8S globulins (vicilins), 11S globulin (legumins)	Thermostable and digestion-stable important primary food allergens in legumes (peanut, soy), tree nuts (hazelnut), capsule fruits, and seeds with limited cross-reactivity within the subfamilies of different species; primary sensitization starts in early childhood and can persist lifelong; high allergen-specific IgE levels are associated with systemic allergic reactions	Ara h 1, 2, and 3 (peanut); Cor a 9, 11, and 14 (hazelnut)

Modified from the I/LA20 Guidance Document from the Clinical Laboratory Standard's Institute. Hamilton RG, Matsson PNJ, Chan S, et al. Analytical performance characteristics, quality assurance and clinical utility of immunological assays for human immunoglobulin E (IgE) antibodies of defined allergen specificities. 3rd ed. I/LA20-A3, International CLSI-Guideline. Wayne, PA: Clinical Laboratory Standards Institute; 2016.

currently in commercial use in the United States have found a heterologous interpolation procedure to be optimal in which allergen-specific IgE antibody response data are interpolated from a total serum IgE calibration curve. This procedure is valid as long as the total IgE calibrators and the patient's allergen-specific IgE antibody levels dilute out in parallel so that parallelism is maintained. The assays report IgE antibody levels in the same units (kUa/L), using internal total IgE calibrators that are cross-verified and

traceable to the World Health Organization (WHO) 11/234 IgE international reference preparation.[29] This calibration system allows interpolation of IgE antibody results from a limit of quantitation of 0.1 kUa/L to 100 kUa/L levels of IgE antibody. In terms of quantitation, at least one of the IgE antibody autoanalyzers (ImmunoCAP) has demonstrated equivalence in which 1 kUa/L of chimeric allergen-specific IgE antibody was shown to be equivalent to 1 kU/L (2.4 ng/mL) of total serum IgE.[30]

Single-Plex, Multiallergen, and Multiplex Assays
The autoanalyzers in common clinical use are single-plex (or monoplex) assays in which one analyte (*e.g.,* IgE anti−cat dander) is measured in a single analysis. In contrast, a multiplex antibody assay allows many specificities of a single antibody isotype (*e.g.,* IgE) to be individually detected and semiquantified in a single analysis. These are distinguished from a multiallergen screening assay, which is a form of single-plex analysis that involves the use of a mix of multiple allergens that is immobilized on the same allergosorbent. The purpose of the multiallergen assay is to simultaneously screen a serum for IgE antibody to a concise number (*e.g.,* 10−15) allergens either of the same allergen source type (*e.g.,* foods: chicken egg, cow's milk, peanut, soybean, cod fish) or diverse sources (*e.g.,* respiratory allergens as an aeroallergen mix: pollen from select trees, grasses, weeds, pet epidermals, dust mites, molds).[31] A qualitative result (positive or negative) is generated, and it serves as an inexpensive and efficient single analysis to assess the general atopic status (IgE positivity) of an individual. One multiaeroallergen screening assay is being used to assess the atopic status (genetic predisposition to produce IgE antibody) of research subjects enrolling in clinical studies of asthma.[32] Clinically, the multiaeroallergen screening assay has a high negative predictive power and thus is used to rule out IgE-mediated allergic disease where the suspicion based on the clinical history is weak.

The availability of unlimited quantities of molecular allergens has made it possible to develop multiplex chip based microarrays for diagnostic allergy confirmatory testing. The first microarray for semiquantification of IgE antibody involved a preactivated glass slide or chip on which 94 purified allergens were each immobilized in triplicate microdot arrays.[33] The present day version of this assay is the immune solid phase allergen chip or ISAC (Thermo Fisher Scientific/Phadia, Uppsala, Sweden) in which 40 μL of serum is applied to a chip that has 112 individual allergenic molecules immobilized.[34] IgE anti−cow's milk components as measured in the multiplex ISAC have agreed well with those obtained in a single-plex autoanalyzer using the same allergen specificities.[35] Other groups have tried alternative multiplexing technologies to detect IgE antibodies that have included immobilizing allergen extracts on chips by using Luminex bead−based suspension arrays, employing nanotechnology biosensors, detecting surface plasmon resonance, and using plates equipped to produce electrical pulse generated chemiluminescence.[35,36]

When selecting a single-plex or multiplex assay format, one must consider their strengths and weaknesses. Single-plex systems have the advantage of greater analytical sensitivity or a lower limit of quantitation, greater precision and accuracy, more established internal and external quality control, and wider global availability of technology. In contrast, multiplex systems provide increased speed of analysis with reduced turn-around times, conservation of sample volume, greater simplicity, and reduced technical and reagent costs.[36]

The quality of allergen-specific IgE antibody results reported from clinical diagnostic allergy laboratories is not uniformly equivalent. In addition to the variability of results for a given serum between assays from different manufacturers as a result of allergen and calibration variance, the positive thresholds used for the same assay by different laboratories varies (*e.g.,* 0.1, 0.35, and 0.7 kUa/L).[37] For this reason, physicians requesting IgE antibody testing bear some responsibilities for determining the quality of the results they receive. In the United States, testing should be performed in a clinical laboratory that is federally licensed for highly complex immunology clinical testing under CLIA-88 (verified by requesting a copy of the federal laboratory license).[38] The requesting physician should inquire about the assay method used, the source of its reagents, and how assays are quality controlled by the laboratory. As part of the formal record, the assay method used in patient analysis should be indicated on the final report.

Competitive IgE Antibody Inhibition Assay
The competitive inhibition format of the IgE antibody assay has been used by researchers, allergen manufacturers, and regulators to determine the relative potency of allergen extracts.[39] One practical research application of the IgE antibody inhibition assay has been as a tool for monitoring the concentration of allergens released into environments (*e.g.,* latex allergen in hospital air[40]; air sampling of airplanes for aerosolized peanut allergen). In the diagnostic allergy laboratory, the competitive IgE antibody inhibition assay has been used analytically to confirm an IgE antibody assay's minimum detectable dose (sensitivity) and nonspecific binding and to document the extent of cross-reactivity by determining the allergen specificity of IgE antibody.[13]

The one clinical application of the IgE antibody inhibition assay has been as an adjunct to define the appropriate therapeutic composition of venoms for patients who have insect-sting allergy with multiple potentially cross-reactive sensitivities and who have elected to receive immunotherapy.[41] Indications for this test include a strong skin reactivity; a high level of serum IgE antibody to yellow jacket venom (YJV) and a weak skin reactivity; or a low level of serum IgE antibody specific for *Polistes* wasp venom (PWV). The structural similarity between *Vespid* and *Polistes* wasp phospholipase A1/B (Ves g 1; Pol a 1) and Antigen 5 (Ves g 5; Pol a 5) frequently produces IgE antibody cross-reactivity. Sera from 305 patients with *Hymenoptera* venom allergy with >2 ng/mL of IgE antibody to YJV and PWV were evaluated in the IgE antibody inhibition assay to document its clinical utility. The diagnostic question for these patients is whether PWV should be included in the venom immunotherapy together with yellow jacket or mixed vespid venom. Using this procedure, the venom-specific IgE antibody inhibition assay identified one-third (36.4%) of subjects with a primary YJV sensitivity who were candidates for exclusion of PWV from their immunotherapy regimen because their IgE anti-PWV was >95% cross-inhibitable with soluble YJV.[41]

More recently, molecular venom allergens may be particularly useful in clarifying whether patients with venom allergies with IgE antibody positivity for two or more distinct venoms (YJV, HBV, and/or PWV) reflect true multiple venom sensitization or whether the observed multiple positivity results from either clinically irrelevant cross-reactive carbohydrate-specific IgE antibodies or common protein epitopes of homologous venom antigens.[42] The important carbohydrate cross-reactive determinant (CCD) in insect venoms involves an α1,3-linked fucose residue that is attached to the innermost N-acetylglucosamine carbohydrate on venom proteins.[43] For YJV and HBV, the known cross-reactive proteins include hyaluronidase (Api m 2, Ves v 2), dipeptidyl peptidase (Api m 5, Ves v 3), and vitellogenin (Api m 12, Ves v 6). IgE antibody cross-reactivity between YJV and PWV is independent of CCD and can occur as a result of common epitopes on homologous antigens: antigen 5 (Ves v 5, Pol d 5) and phospholipase A 1 (Ves v 1 and Pol d 1).[44] Specific IgE antibody measurements against rVes v 5 and rPol d 5 alone were able to aid in differentiating sensitivity against *Vespula* and *Polistes* venoms in some patients. However, Savi et al.[45] concluded that the venom competitive inhibition analysis remains the optimal serological test at present for differentiating between true and cross-reactivity-related dual *Vespula* and

Polistes venom sensitization. Moreover, when rPol d 1 becomes available for testing in parallel with currently available Ves v 1, Ves v 5, and Pol d 5, the effectiveness of molecular allergen–based differentiation of dual *Vespula* and *Polistes* venom sensitization will need to be reassessed.

Clinical Pearls
*Clinical Utility of Immunoglobulin E (IgE)
Anti-Hymenoptera Venom Inhibition Test*

- Useful in identifying venom cross-reactive IgE antibodies and selecting appropriate venoms for immunotherapy.
- One-third of venom-allergic patients with concomitant yellow jacket venom (YJV) and *Polistes* wasp venom (PWV) sensitivity can be treated with YJV alone or mixed vespid venoms, owing to >95% cross-reactive IgE anti-PWV with soluble YJV.

Allergen-Specific IgG

Allergen immunotherapy is known to enhance the production of specific IgG "blocking" antibodies.[46,47] Quantitative measurements of allergen-specific total IgG or IgG subclass antibodies in studies of allergic rhinitis have not generally correlated with the control of clinical symptoms in individual patients. However, clinically successful immunotherapy is almost always accompanied by high serum levels of allergen-specific IgG (typically IgG1 and IgG4) blocking antibodies.[47] Interestingly, despite a decrease to preimmunotherapy baseline levels after 2 years of immunotherapy discontinuation, overall functional inhibitory activity, as measured by an IgE-dependent facilitated allergen binding assay, appears to be maintained.[47] For patients with *Hymenoptera* venom allergy, specific IgG antibody measurements have been used as an indicator of effective immunotherapy. Quantitative venom-specific IgG antibody levels may be useful in individualizing the dose and frequency of injections while maximizing the protective effects. However, their clinical utility may be restricted to the first 4 years of venom immunotherapy.[48] In contrast, the presence or levels of IgG antibodies specific for food antigens have shown no correlation with the results of positive double-blind, placebo-controlled food challenges, and they are not indicated in the diagnostic workup of a patient with suspected food allergy.[20]

Mast-Cell Tryptase

Mast cells have been identified in skin, respiratory, and digestive tract connective tissues and distinguished on the basis of the neutral proteases present in their secretory granules. One group contains only tryptase, whereas the other contains both tryptase and chymase.[49] Mast-cell tryptase (MW 134 kDa) is a serine esterase with four subunits, each having an enzymatically active site. A resting mast cell contains 10–35 picograms (pg) of tryptase that is stored attached to heparin. When dissociated from heparin, it rapidly degrades into its monomers and loses enzymatic activity. As basophils have ~ 500-fold less tryptase compared with mast cells, elevated tryptase levels in serum are considered a relatively specific indicator of mast-cell involvement in a clinical reaction. Unstimulated tissue mast cells continually secrete immature protryptase into the tissue, and it diffuses into the circulation to provide a measure of total mast-cell number. α-Protryptase and β-protryptase represent the bulk of the immature tryptase in nonanaphylactic sera. α-Protryptase remains enzymatically inactive, whereas some of β-protryptase is autoprocessed from the proform within the mast cell into the mature enzyme by a dipeptidase where it is stored in granules.[50] Only upon activation of mast cells are both the pro and mature forms of tryptase secreted in parallel with prestored histamine and newly generated vasoactive mediators. Total tryptase in serum from healthy humans ranges from 1 to 11.4 µg/L (average 3–5 µg/L). Mature tryptase is normally undetectable (<1 µg/L) in serum from healthy individuals who have no history of anaphylaxis during the preceding hours. A noncompetitive two-site fluorescent enzyme immunoassay (Phadia, ImmunoCAP) is available to measure total tryptase in serum. Elevated levels of total tryptase (>11.4 µg/L) can be detected in serum 1–4 hours after the onset of systemic anaphylaxis with hypotension. Baseline levels of >20 µg/L are detected in most individuals with systemic mastocytosis.[50] Recommended serum collection times for tryptase quantification range from 30 minutes to 4 hours after the onset of an acute event. Because serological tests for mature tryptase are not widely available, it is important to compare an acute event total tryptase level (within 4 hours) with a baseline total tryptase 24 hours after all signs and symptoms of the event have subsided.[50] Postmortem specimens are often difficult to analyze for tryptase because of high viscosity related to gross hemolysis. However, reported mature tryptase levels in postmortem cases of fatal anaphylaxis have ranged from 12 to 150 µg/L in all nine fatalities caused by *Hymenoptera* venom and in six of eight food-induced fatalities.[51] The frequency of a severe reaction to venom from a *Hymenoptera* sting increases significantly with higher serum baseline total tryptase concentrations.[52,53] The clinical indications for and diagnostic value of tryptase as a marker of anaphylaxis and mastocytosis are reviewed elsewhere.[52]

Basophil Mediator Release Assays

There are a number of diagnostic assays for sensitization that use the basophil as the indicator modality. Some assays monitor the magnitude of mediator release from basophils, and others assess the degree of cell surface marker expression following exposure to allergen.

Histamine Release Assay

The potent vasoactive mediator histamine is stored in cytoplasmic granules of basophilic leukocytes and mast cells. It is released along with other mediators of inflammation in response to both immunological and nonimmunological stimuli.[54] The basophil histamine release (BHR) assay has been particularly useful as a quantitative assay of allergen potency and as an *in vitro* model for the study of triggering mechanisms of mediator release from basophils. In its most basic form, peripheral blood leukocytes are isolated from a donor and incubated with varying concentrations (*e.g.*, 3- to 10-fold dilutions) of allergen extract or anti-human IgE as a positive control. Histamine release is complete within 30 minutes, and then histamine in the supernatant is measured by enzymatic, radiometric, or spectrophotofluorometric techniques.[55] Details of the BHR assay are given elsewhere.[54,56]

Patient sensitivity for a given allergen can be determined with a positive BHR test. The results are highly correlated with those determined by skin testing[55] and bronchoprovocation.[57] Although the BHR test has been almost exclusively used in research laboratories because of its expense, time-consuming nature, and the need for fresh blood (<24 hours old), it can be successfully applied to the clinical diagnosis of allergic disease in selected cases. Its results parallel those of other IgE antibody tests. BHR has also been a useful tool for clarifying discrepancies between skin test and serological IgE antibody test results.

Leukotriene C4 Release Assay

An assay method for measuring leukotriene C4 (LTC4) released from allergen-activated basophils has been reported as the cellular antigen stimulation test (CAST)-enzyme-linked immunosorbent assay (ELISA).[58] The LTC4 assay is designed for use with either whole blood preparations or washed leukocytes. Using dust mite, food, *Hymenoptera* venoms,[59] and drugs as challenge allergens, the observed diagnostic sensitivity of the CAST compared with the combination of a clinical history and skin test ranged from 18% with aspirin and 50–85% for selected food allergens.[60] The reported diagnostic specificity of the CAST in the same studies ranged from 67% to 100%. These data indicate that the CAST assay is not sufficiently sensitive for effective clinical use in the diagnosis of IgE-mediated sensitivities to β-lactam or nonsteroidal antiinflammatory drugs (NSAIDs). Its utility in the diagnosis of sensitization to other allergen specificities appears more promising, but further documentation involving clinical studies is required.

Utility of Mediator Release Assays as Diagnostic Tests

Despite their unquestioned value as research methods, the basophil histamine and LTC4 release assays are rarely used clinically in the routine diagnosis of human allergic disease, and it is unlikely that this trend will change in the foreseeable future.

Flow Cytometry Basophil Activation Assays

In the late 1990s, basophils were shown to upregulate the expression of a number of surface proteins (*e.g.*, CD45, CD63, CD69, and CD203c) when activated by allergen.[60–62] CD63 is a member of the transmembrane-4 superfamily that is expressed on basophils, mast cells, macrophages, and platelets.[60,61] In resting basophils from individuals without atopia and allergies, CD63 is attached to intracytoplasmic granules. Activated IgE-sensitized basophils express a high density of CD63 on their surface. By quantifying ∼500 basophils with gated flow cytometry, the percentage of activated basophils can be identified, after correcting for spontaneous CD63 expression. A variety of criteria are used to identify an allergen-induced positive response, such as a stimulation index (allergen-induced/basal ratio) >2.

One confounding variable in this analysis is the adherence of CD63-expressing platelets in basophil preparations that can sometimes generate false-positive results.

The flow assay stimulation test (FAST), which is also referred to as the basophil activation test (BAT) or BasoTest, uses CD63 as a marker for activation. Its performance was evaluated by using minor determinant mixture, benzyl penicilloyl polylysine, penicillin, ampicillin, amoxicillin, and cephalosporin as stimulating antigens.[62,67] Subjects (n = 58) with a history of immediate-type reactions to β-lactam antibiotics or nonallergic controls (n = 30) were evaluated in the CD63 FAST/BAT and Phadia ImmunoCAP system for drug-specific IgE levels. Relative to the clinical history, the CD63 FAST/BAT displayed a diagnostic sensitivity and specificity of 50% and 93%, respectively. Diagnostic sensitivity was marginally increased to 66% by simultaneously using the drug-specific IgE antibody serology result. The study concluded that the CD63 basophil activation test could be helpful in supporting the diagnosis of IgE-mediated allergy to β-lactam drugs when used in conjunction with an additional diagnostic test, such as IgE antibody serology.[63]

CD203c (also known as *neural cell surface differentiation antigen, E-NIPP3 PD-1β, 97A6, B10,* and *gp130rb13−6*) is a member of the ectonucleotide pyrophosphate phosphodiesterase (E-NPP) family.[64] It is expressed only on IgE-bearing basophils, mast cells, and their progenitors and is upregulated after activation of IgE-sensitized basophils with allergen or anti-IgE in a manner similar to CD63. The CD203c-based flow assay is performed in a manner analogous to the CD63-based assay. Its advantage over CD63 is its restricted expression on basophils in peripheral blood, which minimizes concern about the adherence of platelets that may produce false-positive CD63 results. Additionally, there is no need for the use of an additional fluorescent anti-IgE reagent to gate the basophils. Basophil activation as determined by CD203c expression was studied in patients with allergy to *Hymenoptera* venom and healthy controls in which their basophils were activated with anti-IgE or bee/*Vespid* venoms.[65] Fifteen minutes after stimulation, basophils from 15 wasp-sensitized patients upregulated CD203c expression from 4.2-fold to 13.5-fold. Moreover, basophils from six patients with honeybee venom allergy upregulated CD203c by a mean of 8.3-fold. The study concluded that the CD203c-based flow assay could confirm the presence of venom-specific IgE antibody on basophils in 20 of 22 patients (91%) with a clinical history of and skin test positivity to venom allergy. One false-positive result was observed among 13 healthy controls with a negative result on the skin test.

Diagnostic Utility of Basophil Activation Flow Cytometric Assays

The utility of basophil activation flow cytometric assays is limited by a number of technical concerns.[63,66] First, endotoxin-free whole blood must be received within 24 hours by the laboratory, where it can be processed by skilled technologists. Second, the blood is preincubated with stimulation buffer often containing IL-3, which primes basophils. It is unclear what effect IL-3 has on altering mediator release or CD63/CD203c upregulation, and thus false-positive mediator release and/or biomarker surface expression are potential concerns. Third, varying concentrations of crude allergen extract or recombinant allergen or anti-IgE are incubated with the cell preparation. Unfortunately, crude extracts lack potency estimates and can often be cytotoxic. Thus each stimulating allergen needs to be prequalified with basophils from well-characterized patients before use. Fourth, criteria for defining positive assay results vary among the laboratories performing the test, and stimulating allergen preparations from even the same manufacturer can have variable potency. Fifth, there is a concern about false-positive results related to platelet adherence on basophils in the CD63 based BAT assay. Possibly most important, when the performance characteristics were directly compared in clinical studies to puncture skin test results, the diagnostic sensitivity and specificity of the flow-cytometric analysis of in vitro allergen-activated basophils were less than optimal. For these reasons, cell-based cytometric methods will most likely remain useful research techniques for the investigation of allergic disease, but they will have limited application to clinical diagnosis.

On the Horizon

New trends in laboratory methodology for the assessment of human allergic diseases include the following:

- Although there is a transition from the use of crude allergen extracts to allergenic components in immunoglobulin E (IgE) antibody serological assays, extracts will remain the principal allergen reagent source for the foreseeable future because of their comprehensive nature.
- Multiplexing platforms are being increasingly developed to allow rapid simultaneous detection of IgE antibodies to many allergenic components using microliter quantities of serum; however, due to their semiquantitative nature, fixed panel of specificities, and lower analytical sensitivity, single-plex assays will remain the most cost-effective and widely used assay format for the foreseeable future.

- Qualitative "point of care" IgE antibody assays to rapidly assess sensitization to aeroallergens during the patient's visit will be slow to be adopted because of their limited/fixed allergen menus, lower diagnostic sensitivity, and concern about potential patient misinterpretation of results.

REFERENCES

1. Prausnitz C, Kustner H. Studine uber die Ueberemfindlichkeil. *Zentralbl Bakteriol Mikrobiol Hyg.* 1921;86:160 [in German].
2. Ishizaka K, Ishizaka T. Physiochemical properties of reaginic antibody. I. Association of reaginic activity with an immunoglobulin other than gamma A or gamma G globulin. *J Allergy.* 1967;37:169.
3. Johansson SGO. Raised levels of a new immunoglobulin class (IgND) in asthma. *Lancet.* 1967;2:951.
4. Hamilton RG. The science behind the discovery of IgE. *J Allergy Clin Immunol.* 2005;115:648.
5. Hamilton RG. Human immunoglobulins. In: O'Gorman MRG, Donnenberg AD, eds. *Handbook of Human Immunology.* 2nd ed. Boca Raton, FL: CRC Press; 2008: 63−106.
6. Barbee RA, Halomen M, Lebowitz M, et al. Distribution of IgE in a community population sample: correlations with age, sex and allergen skin test reactivity. *J Allergy Clin Immunol.* 1981;68:106.
7. Kleine-Tebbe J, Poulsen LK, Hamilton RG. Quality management in IgE-based allergy diagnostics. *J Lab Med.* 2016;40:81−96.
8. Wittig HJ, Belloit J, DeFillippi I, et al. Age-related serum IgE levels in healthy subjects and in patients with allergic disease. *J Allergy Clin Immunol.* 1980;66:305.
9. Dati F, Ringel KP. Reference values for serum IgE in healthy nonatopic children and adults. *Clin Chem.* 1982;28:1556.
10. Lin H, Boesel KM, Griffith DT, et al. Omalizumab rapidly decreases nasal allergic response and FcεR1 on basophils. *J Allergy Clin Immunol.* 2004;113:297.
11. Saini SS, Bindslev-Jensen C, Maurer M, et al. Efficacy and safety of omalizumab in patients with chronic idiopathic/spontaneous urticaria who remain symptomatic on H1 antihistamines: a randomized, placebo-controlled study. *J Invest Dermatol.* 2015;135:67−75.
12. Wide L, Bennich H, Johansson SGO. Diagnosis by an in vitro test for allergen specific antibodies. *Lancet.* 1967;2:1105.
13. Hamilton RG, Matsson PNJ, Chan S, et al. *Analytical Performance Characteristics, Quality Assurance and Clinical Utility of Immunological Assays for Human Immunoglobulin E (IgE) Antibodies of Defined Allergen Specificities.* 3rd ed. I/LA20−A3, International CLSI-Guideline. Wayne, PA: Clinical Laboratory Standards Institute; 2016.
14. Hamilton RG, Oppenheimer J. Serological IgE analyses in the diagnostic algorithm for allergic disease. *J Allergy Clin Immunol Pract.* 2015;3:833−840.

15. Yunginger JW, Ahlstedt S, Eggleston PA, et al. Quantitative IgE antibody assays in allergic diseases. *J Allergy Clin Immunol.* 2000;105:1077.

16. Adkinson Jr NF, Hamilton RG. Clinical history-driven diagnosis of allergic diseases: utilizing in vitro IgE testing. *J Allergy Clin Immunol Pract.* 2015;3:871–876.

17. Hamilton RG. Allergic sensitization is a key risk factor for but not synonymous with allergic disease. *J Allergy Clin Immunol.* 2014;134:360–361.

18. Hamilton RG. Diagnostic in vivo and in vitro methods in insect allergy. In: Freeman T, Tracy J, eds. *Stinging Insect Allergy: A Clinician's Guide.* NY: Springer Science; 2017:85–99.

19. Hamilton RG. Assessment of human allergic diseases. In: Rich RR, et al., eds. *Clinical Immunology: Principles and Practice.* 5th ed. Elsevier; 2019:1283.

20. Stapel SO, Asero R, Ballmer-Weber BK, et al. Testing for IgG4 against foods is not recommended as a diagnostic tool: EAACI Task Force Report. *Allergy.* 2008;63:793–796.

21. Participants summary report. *College of American pathologists, diagnostic allergy (SE) survey, Cycle B.* Northfield, IL: College of American Pathologists; 2015.

22. Chang TW, Davis FM, Sun NC, et al. Monoclonal antibodies specific for human IgE producing B cells: a potential therapeutic for IgE mediated allergic diseases. *Biotechnology (NY).* 1990;8:122–126.

23. Hamilton RG. Accuracy of US Food and Drug Administration cleared IgE antibody assays in the presence of anti-IgE (omalizumab). *J Allergy Clin Immunol.* 2006;117:759–766.

24. Baker DL, Peng K, Cheu M, et al. Evaluation of two commercial omalizumab/free IgE immunoassays: implications for use during therapy. *Curr Med Res Opin.* 2014;30:913–922.

25. Hamilton RG. Monitoring allergic patients on omalizumab with free and total serum IgE measurements. *J Allergy Clin Immunol Pract.* 2016;4:366–368.

26. Radauer C, Bublin M, Wagner S, et al. Allergens are distributed into few protein families and possess a restricted number of biochemical functions. *J Allergy Clin Immunol.* 2008;121:847–852.

27. Kleine-Tebbe J, Matricardi PM, Hamilton RG. Allergy work-up including component-resolved diagnosis: how to make allergen-specific immunotherapy more specific. *Immunol Allergy Clin North Am.* 2016;36:191–203.

28. European Academy of Asthma Allergy and Clinical Immunology working group. Matricardi P, Kleine-Tebbe J, Ollert M, et al, editors. Handbook on molecular allergology. *Pediatr Allergy Immunol.* 2016;23:1–250.

29. Thorpe S, Heath A, Fox B, et al. The 3rd international standard for serum IgE: international collaborative study to evaluate a candidate preparation. *Clin Chem Lab Med.* 2014;52:1283–1289.

30. Kober A, Perborn H. Quantitation of mouse-human chimeric allergen-specific IgE antibodies with ImmunoCAP technology. *J Allergy Clin Immunol.* 2006;117:S219, [Abstract 845].

31. Merrett J, Merrett TG. Phadiatop—a novel antibody screening test. *Clin Allergy.* 1987;17:409–416.

32. Szefler SJ, Wenzel S, Brown R, et al. Asthma outcomes: biomarker. *J Allergy Clin Immunol.* 2012;129:S9–23.

33. Hiller R, Laffer S, Harwanegg C, et al. Microarrayed allergen molecules: diagnostic gatekeepers for allergy treatment. *FASEB J.* 2002;16:414–416.

34. Martínez-Aranguren R, Lizaso MT, Goikoetxea MJ, et al. Is the determination of specific IgE against components using ISAC 112 a reproducible technique? *PLoS ONE.* 2014;9:e88394.

35. Chapman MD, Wuenschmann S, King E, et al. Technological innovations for high-throughput approaches to in vitro allergy diagnosis. *Curr Allergy Asthma Rep.* 2015;15:36.

36. Hamilton RG, Kleine-Tebbe J. Methods for IgE antibody testing: singleplex and multiplex assays. In: Matricardi P, Kleine-Tebbe J, Ollert M, et al., eds. *Handbook on Molecular Allergology. Pediatr Allergy Immunology.* 2016;23:1–250.

37. Hamilton RG. Clinical laboratories worldwide need to report IgE antibody results on clinical specimens as analytical results and not use differential positive thresholds. *J Allergy Clin Immunol.* 2015;136:811–812, 9.

38. Hamilton RG. Responsibility for quality IgE antibody results rests ultimately with the referring physician. *Ann Allergy Asthma Immunol.* 2001;86:353–354.

39. Nordlee JA, Taylor SL, Jones RT, et al. Allergenicity of various peanut products as determined by RAST inhibition. *J Allergy Clin Immunol.* 1981;68:376–382.

40. Charous BL, Schuenemann PJ, Swanson MC. Passive dispersion of latex aeroallergen in a healthcare facility. *Ann Allergy Asthma Immunol.* 2000;85:285–290.

41. Hamilton RG, Wisenauer JA, Golden DB, et al. Selection of *Hymenoptera* venoms for immunotherapy based on patient's IgE antibody cross-reactivity. *J Allergy Clin Immunol.* 1993;92:651.

42. Muller UR, Johansen N, Petersen AB, et al. *Hymenoptera* venom allergy: analysis of double positivity to honey bee and *Vespula* venom by estimation of IgE antibodies to species-specific major allergens Api m1 and Ves v5. *Allergy.* 2009;64:543–548.

43. Ollert M, Blank S. Anaphylaxis to insect venom allergens: role of molecular diagnostics. *Curr Allergy Asthma Rep.* 2015;15:26.

44. Caruso B, Bonadonna P, Bovo C, et al. Wasp venom allergy screening with recombinant allergen testing. Diagnostic performance of rPol d 5 and rVes v 5 for differentiating sensitization to *Vespula* and *Polistes* subspecies. *Clin Chim Acta.* 2016;435:170–173.

45. Savi E, Peveri S, Makri E, et al. Comparing the ability of molecular diagnosis and CAP-inhibition in identifying the really causative venom in patients with positive tests to *Vespula* and *Polistes* species. *Clin Mol Allergy.* 2016;14:3.

46. Sobotka AK, Valentine MD, Ishizaka K, et al. Measurement of IgG-blocking antibodies: development and application of a radioimmunoassay. *J Immunol.* 1976;117:84–90.

47. James LK, Shamji MH, Walker SM, et al. Long-term tolerance after allergen immunotherapy is accompanied by selective persistence of blocking antibodies. *J Allergy Clin Immunol.* 2011;127:509–516.

48. Golden DBK, Lawrence ID, Hamilton RG, et al. Clinical correlation of the venom-specific IgG antibody level

during maintenance venom immunotherapy. *J Allergy Clin Immunol.* 1992;90:386−391.

49. Craig CS, Schwartz LB. Tryptase and chymase: markers of distinct types of human mast cells. *Immunol Res.* 1989;8:130.

50. Sprung J, Weingarten TN, Schwartz LB. Presence or absence of elevated acute total serum tryptase by itself is not a definitive marker for an allergic reaction. *Anesthesiology.* 2015;122:713−714.

51. Yunginger JW, Nelson DR, Squillace DL, et al. Laboratory investigation of deaths due to anaphylaxis. *J Forensic Sci.* 1991;35:857−865.

52. Miller JS, Schwartz LB. Tryptase levels as an indication of mast cell activation in a patient with Hymenoptera anaphylaxis and mastocytosis. *N Engl J Med.* 1987;316:1622.

53. Ruëff F, Przybilla B, Biló MB, et al. Predictors of severe systemic anaphylactic reactions in patients with Hymenoptera venom allergy: importance of baseline serum tryptase-a study of the EAACI Interest Group on Insect Venom Hypersensitivity. *J Allergy Clin Immunol.* 2009;124:1047.

54. Lichtenstein LM, Osler AG. Studies on the mechanisms of hypersensitivity phenomenon. IX. Histamine release from human leukocytes by ragweed pollen. *J Exp Med.* 1964; 120:507.

55. Siraganian RP. Automated histamine analysis for in vitro allergy testing. II. Correlation of skin test results with in vitro whole blood histamine release in 82 patients. *J Allergy Clin Immunol.* 1977;59:214.

56. Ito K, Sato S, Urisu A, et al. An evaluation of spontaneous histamine release and the low responders in a basophil histamine release test. *Arerugi.* 2016;65:48−56.

57. Wegner F, Hockamp R, Rutschke A, et al. Superiority of the histamine release test above case history, prick test and radioallergosorbent test in predicting bronchial reactivity to the house dust mite in asthmatic children. *Klin Wochenschr.* 1983;61:43.

58. de Weck AL. Cellular allergen stimulation test (CAST): a new dimension in allergy diagnostics. *ACI News.* 1993;1: 9−14.

59. Maly FE, Marti-Wyss S, Blumber S, et al. Mononuclear blood cell sulpholeukotriene generation in the presence of interleukin 3 and whole blood histamine release in honeybee and yellow jacket venom allergy. *J Invest Allergy Clin Immunol.* 1997;7:217−224.

60. Moneret-Vautrin DA, Sainte-Laudy J, Kanny G, et al. Human basophil activation as measured by CD63 expression and LTC4 release in IgE-mediated food allergy. *Ann Allergy Asthma Immunol.* 1999;82:33.

61. Bochner BS, Sterbinsky SA, Saini SA, et al. Studies of cell adhesion and flow cytometric analyses of degranulation, surface phenotype and viability using human eosinophils, basophils and mast cells. *Methods.* 1997;13: 61−68.

62. Sanz ML, Gamboa PM, Antepara I. Flow cytometric basophil activation test by detection of CD63 expression in patients with immediate-type reactions to beta lactam antibiotics. *Clin Exp Allergy.* 2002;32:277−286.

63. Mangodt EA, Van Gasse AL, Decuyper I, et al. In vitro diagnosis of immediate drug hypersensitivity: should we go with the flow? [Review]. *Int Arch Allergy Immunol.* 2015; 168:3−12.

64. Buhring HJ, Sieffert M, Giesert C. The basophil activation marker defined by antigen 97A6 is identical to ectonucleotide pyrophosphate/ phosphodiesterase 3. *Blood.* 2001;97: 3303−3305.

65. Platz I, Binder M, Marxer A, et al. Hymenoptera venom induced up regulation of basophil activation marker ecto-nucleotide pyrophosphatase/phosphoesterase 3 (E-NNP3, CD203c) in sensitized individuals. *Int Arch Allergy Immunol.* 2001;126:335−342.

66. Ebo DG, Hagendorens MM, Bridts CH, et al. In vitro allergy diagnosis: should we follow the flow? [Review]. *Clin Exp Allergy.* 2004;34:332−339.

67. Hoffmann HJ, Santos AF, Mayorga C, et al. The clinical utility of basophil activation testing in diagnosis and monitoring of allergic disease. *Allergy.* 2015;70: 1393−1405.

CHAPTER 6

Laboratory Evaluation of Suspected Immunodeficiency

JAVIER CHINEN • MARY E. PAUL • WILLIAM T. SHEARER

Clinical immunologists are often consulted to evaluate patients for suspected immune defects, usually because such patients have an unusual frequency or severity of infectious illnesses. Indeed, immunodeficiency presents with increased susceptibility to infection but may also manifest with conditions that reflect dysregulation of the immune response, such as allergies, autoimmunity, or lymphoproliferation. Prompt diagnosis is essential to reduce the risk of organ damage caused by preventable severe infections. Primary immunodeficiencies (PIDs) are congenital diseases that might affect any aspect of the immune response and are often diagnosed in childhood. Examples of PIDs include severe combined immune deficiencies (SCIDs), complete DiGeorge syndrome, and chronic granulomatous disease (CGD). In contrast to PIDs, secondary immunodeficiencies present at any age, as a result of a wide variety of factors that affect the immune function, such as environmental factors, metabolic disease, anatomical abnormalities, or infectious agents. The most known and significant secondary immunodeficiency is caused by human immunodeficiency virus (HIV). The assessment of a patient for PID should include history and physical examination to direct immunology laboratory testing to confirm a diagnosis.

EPIDEMIOLOGY—PRIMARY IMMUNODEFICIENCIES ARE NOT UNCOMMON

Estimates of the incidence of PIDs or congenital immunodeficiencies vary from selective immunoglobulin A (IgA) deficiency, a relatively common condition (1/223−1/1000 people),[1] to the less common SCID. Recent analysis from 11 state programs established for universal newborn screening for T-cell deficiencies in the United States reported an incidence of SCID of 1/58 000 live births, comparable with childhood leukemia.[2] A household-based telephone survey suggested that 1 in 1200 persons in the United States has been diagnosed with a PID.[3] The minimal incidence of primary immunodeficiencies in the United Kingdom has been estimated at 1 per 13,157 births.[4] Although significant progress has been made to stop the acquired immunodeficiency syndrome (AIDS) epidemic, HIV infection continues to be the most prevalent cause of immunodeficiency worldwide, with an estimated 36.9 million people living with HIV.[5]

PRIMARY VERSUS SECONDARY IMMUNODEFICIENCY

> **Key Concepts**
> *Secondary Immunodeficiencies*
>
> Immunodeficiency is often secondary or transient, caused by nonimmune factors, including the following:
> - Chronic use of high-dose steroids, or other immunosuppressive medications
> - Previous use of monoclonal antibodies (mAbs), such as rituximab (anti-CD20)
> - Protein losses via the gastrointestinal or urinary tract
> - Severe illness requiring critical care
> - Malnutrition
> - Human immunodeficiency virus (HIV) infection

Because of their common occurrence, acquired and nonimmunological causes for recurrent infections should be first considered in the differential diagnosis of the patient with a suspected immune disorder. Acquired conditions that might increase the frequency of infections include allergic inflammation, HIV infection, and the use of immunosuppressive drugs. Patients presenting with low Ig levels might have loss

Core Laboratory Technologies in Clinical Immunology. https://doi.org/10.1016/B978-0-323-66149-2.00006-2

of antibodies as a result of a protein-losing enteropathy, nephropathy, or massive protein loss through skin, such as in severe eczema or burns.[6] Secondary immunodeficiency can also result from other conditions affecting cell metabolism (*e.g.,* malnutrition, diabetes mellitus, and sickle cell anemia) or could be secondary to predictable or idiopathic adverse effects of drugs.

EVALUATING PATIENTS FOR IMMUNODEFICIENCY

The evaluation of patients for immunodeficiency is based on a careful assessment of patient history and physical examination, with limited initial laboratory testing (Fig. 6.1). The limitations of available clinically validated testing need to be considered, as such tests may not be sensitive or specific to identify uncommon immune defects, such as impairments in phagocyte function other than oxidative burst deficiency. The medical history and initial laboratory testing often provide clues that suggest a specific immune disorder, and the examination of specific component of the immune response or a diagnostic test for specific immunodeficiencies may be indicated (Table 6.1). For example, an increased frequency of infections affecting only the respiratory tract and caused by encapsulated bacteria direct the exploration to defects in humoral immunity and complement; in contrast, a history of *Aspergillus* pneumonia would suggest testing for neutropenia and neutrophil oxidative defect. According to the complexity of the illness, clinical immunologists may recommend an initial exploration of one or all of the major components of the immune system: lymphocyte subset distribution, antibody responses, T-cell function, phagocyte oxidative burst, and the complement system.

LABORATORY TESTING FOR IMMUNE FUNCTION

Results from commonly ordered tests might provide a great deal of information about the immune system. The complete blood count (CBC) with differential and platelet determination is ordered to quantitate the total white blood cell (WBC) count and total numbers of neutrophils, lymphocytes, eosinophils, and platelets. Age-specific ranges should be used to determine abnormal cell counts (Appendix 2). Leukocytosis, neutropenia, lymphopenia, and abnormalities in WBC morphology can be detected from this test. Persistent neutrophilia might suggest leukocyte adhesion deficiency (LAD). Anemia may be present in children with chronic disease. Platelet counts may be abnormally low in children with poor bone marrow function or autoimmune disease, and platelets will be reduced in number and morphologically small in children with Wiscott-Aldrich syndrome (WAS). Chemistry panels, including serum liver enzymes levels, might suggest organ compromise as a result of infections or autoimmunity associated with immunodeficiency. Low protein serum levels suggest malnutrition and conditions associated with protein losses, which may cause hypogammaglobulinemia. Examination of the posteroanterior and lateral chest radiographs to look for a thymic shadow can be helpful because its absence is associated with impaired T-cell development. This is especially useful in infants because the thymus mass normally involutes with age. In addition, the thymus may shrink in response to such stresses as surgery, infection, or high-dose steroid treatment.

HIV infection can be ruled out by screening with measurement of anti-HIV antibodies, by the

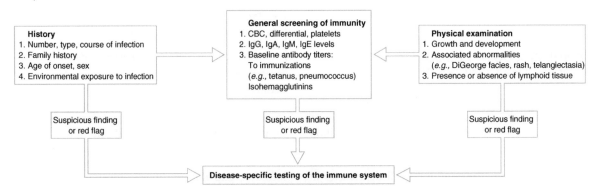

FIG. 6.1 Evaluation of Immunity in a Patient for Immunodeficiency. In addition to a careful history and physical examination, the outlined laboratory tests provide an adequate screen of immunity in a patient with no specific findings.

TABLE 6.1
Correlation of Clinical and Laboratory Findings for the Diagnosis of Immunodeficiencies

	T-Cell Function Defect	Antibody Defect	Granulocyte Defect	Complement Defect	IFN-γ/IL-12 Defect
Recurrent or severe bacterial infections	X	X	X (catalase-positive)	X (encapsulated bacteria)	
Systemic mycobacterial infections	X				X
Recurrent or severe viral infections	X	X	X		X
Invasive fungal infections	X		X		
Opportunistic infections	X		X		X
Failure to thrive	X	X	X		
Autoimmunity	X	X	X	X	
Lymphoma	X	X (CVID)			

CVID, common variable immunodeficiency; *IFN*, interferon; *IL*, interleukin.

enzyme-linked immunosorbent assay (ELISA) or the rapid HIV test. In those individuals with suspected humoral immunity defect and in children younger than 18 months of age, a polymerase chain reaction (PCR)–based test to detect HIV viremia should be performed to avoid false-negative results and confounding maternal anti-HIV antibodies, respectively.

Immunology Testing

Key Concepts
Screening Tests for Suspected Immunodeficiency

- Evaluation for neutropenia, lymphopenia, thrombocytopenia, and/or small platelets
- Immunoglobulin levels and specific antibodies to childhood immunizations
- Lateral chest radiography in infants for thymus shadow
- Consider flow cytometry to quantify T cells, T-cell subsets, B cells, and natural killer (NK) cells (especially in infants)
- Measurement of CH50 activity
- Test for oxidative burst in phagocytes

Specific immunological testing is guided by clues obtained from the history and physical examination and common screening laboratory tests.

Serum Immunoglobulin Levels

The levels of IgG, IgA, IgE, and IgM can be measured in serum. The IgA level is especially helpful in that it is low in all permanent types of agammaglobulinemia and in selective IgA deficiency. IgE level measurement is of significance for the diagnosis of hyper-IgE syndromes. Serum IgG subclass levels can be determined. However, rather than using IgG subclass levels to screen for immunodeficiency, they are best utilized when patients have clinical conditions associated with specific antibody deficiencies but normal total IgG levels. In some of these patients, an IgG subclass deficiency, particularly IgG2 and IgG3 deficiencies, might be present. IgG2 subclass deficiency has been linked with selective IgA deficiency and deficiency of antipolysaccharide antibodies. IgA subclass low levels, IgA1, IgA2, have not been associated with a specific immune defect, and there is no validity for measuring these. The variation of normal ranges of human serum Igs with age is an important consideration in children, since IgA and IgG subclass levels may not reach normal adult reference ranges until 6 years of age.[1]

B-Cell Function: Specific Antibody Production

To properly assess B-cell function, specific antibody production must be measured. Patients with normal Ig and Ig subclass levels might exhibit deficient antigen-dependent antibody responses. An initial screen of antibody production may involve the quantification of isohemagglutinins. Isohemagglutinins occur in all individuals except those with blood type AB; isohemagglutinins are natural IgM antibodies to polysaccharide blood group antigens A and/or B, which are not expressed in the red blood cells (RBCs) of the patient tested. Individuals form isohemagglutinins as a result of environmental exposure to ubiquitous antigens that share epitopes with blood antigens. Children less than 1 year of age do not reliably have measurable serum isohemagglutinins because of the limited exposure to the environment. A patient with blood type A should have anti-B IgM; patients with blood type B should have anti-A IgM; and patients with blood type O should have both anti-A and anti-B IgM. These antibodies are normally present in titers greater than 1:10; individuals with poor antibody production may have low or absent titers. Specific IgG antibody production can be measured following immunization with protein antigens, such as toxoids derived from *Tetanus* and *Diphtheria* organisms, and polysaccharide antigens, such as those produced by pneumococci and *Haemophilus influenzae*. For pneumococcal immunization, there are two vaccines that need to be differentiated. The conjugated vaccine containing 13 pneumococcal serotypes (PCV13, Wyeth) is currently included in the universal schedule of immunizations for infants and toddlers and induces a robust, T cell–dependent immune response. The unconjugated 23-valent pneumococcal polysaccharide vaccine (Pneumovax23, Merck) is available for immunization to adults and children aged 2 years and older. The immune response for this vaccine is considered less dependent on T cells and less lasting than the conjugated vaccine. The pneumococcal antigen challenge using the unconjugated vaccine is not recommended for children under 2 years of age because there has been concern that healthy children do not reliably respond to the unconjugated pneumococcal antigen at this age. However, this view has been challenged by data showing that 1-year-old children produce normal antibody responses to this unconjugated vaccine.[7,8] Normal antibody responses are usually demonstrated with an over twofold rise in specific antibody levels within 2–3 weeks for protein antigens and within 4–6 weeks for polysaccharide antigens.[9] Patients with agammaglobulinemia are expected not to produce antibody responses, whereas others, such as those with IgG2 subclass deficiency and normal levels of total IgG, may only have difficulty with antibody production following immunization with polysaccharide antigens. Patients with selective IgA deficiency, alone or with transient hypogammaglobulinemia of infancy, have

normal specific IgG antibody production, by definition. The pneumococcal serotypes included in the current conjugated antipneumococcal vaccine, serotypes 1, 3, 4, 5, 6A, 6B, 7F, 9V, 14, 18C, 19A, 19F, and 23F, were estimated to be responsible for approximately 90% of invasive pneumococcal disease in children less than 5 years of age worldwide.[10] Previous immunization with the conjugate vaccine does not preclude use of the unconjugated pneumococcal polysaccharide vaccine. The 23-valent polysaccharide vaccine provides the potential for stimulation and measurement of a protective immune response to additional 11 serotypes (2, 8, 9N, 10A, 11A, 12F, 15B, 17F, 20, 22F, 33F) not included in the conjugated vaccine. Testing for antibodies against serotypes not included in the two vaccines and comparing the antibody titers in the pre- and postimmunization blood samples helps in the assessment of specific increase of antiserotype antibody titers as a response to the vaccine administration.

Evaluation of Cellular Immunity

Lymphocyte subset enumeration. Quantitation of B- and T-cell subsets narrows the differential diagnosis and provides evidence for the diagnosis of combined, cellular, or antibody immunodeficiency. Both T and B cells can be identified and labeled by using flow cytometry and fluorescent monoclonal antibodies (mAbs). T-cell enumeration involves the use of a pan-T-cell mAb specific for CD3. The CD4 marker serves as identification for T-helper (Th) cells. CD8 marker characterizes cytotoxic T cells. B cells can be identified by using mAbs against the cell surface markers CD19 or CD20. Natural killer (NK) cells can be identified by using mAbs against CD16 and CD56. Specialized clinical laboratories are available to measure lymphocyte markers of importance to specific diseases; for instance, the proportion of αβ T-cell receptor (αβTCR) and γδTCR double-negative CD3$^+$ T cells is of relevance in the diagnosis of autoimmune lymphoproliferative syndrome (ALPS). T cell subsets can be characterized as naïve or activated based on the expression of CD45RA and CD45RO antigens.

B-cell subset panels and NK-cell subset panels. These panels have been designed to characterize the maturation stage of these cells and provide support for the diagnosis of an immunodeficiency. For example, the proportion of class-switched B cells has a predictive value for autoimmune and granulomatous complications in common variable immunodeficiency.

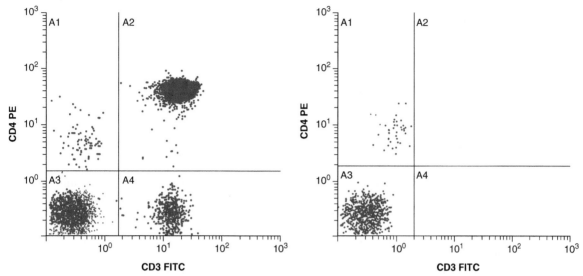

FIG. 6.2 Histograms of Fluorescently Stained Lymphocytes. The quadrant of interest, A2, shows lymphocytes that are positive for labeling with both fluorescein isothiocyanate (FITC)–tagged monoclonal antibodies specific for CD3 and phycoerythrin (PE)–tagged monoclonal antibodies (mAbs) specific for CD4. The histogram on the left shows normal fluorescence as a result of CD4 T lymphocytes present in quadrant A2. The histogram on the right shows absence of CD4 T lymphocytes in an infant with SCID.

In flow cytometry, the fluorescence intensity corresponding to cells labeled with each specific antibody is obtained (Fig. 6.2) and the percentage of the specific lymphocyte subset can be estimated. A reference range is available for each subset defining normal values as those whose values fall between the 5th and 95th percentages for this population. Separate ranges should be used for children because infants and children generally have higher absolute numbers of T-cell subsets and higher percentages of CD4 T cells (Fig. 6.3 and Appendix 2). Nonimmune factors, such as age, gender, and adrenocorticoid levels, influence the expression of blood lymphocyte subset populations. Therefore interpretation of lymphocyte phenotyping should take into consideration the clinical status of the patient. For example, transient moderate lymphopenia with predominance of T cells and NK cells might be seen in patients admitted to intensive care units. HIV infection causes progressive depletion of CD4 T cells. These abnormalities resolve when the patient's condition improves.

Lymphocyte functional analysis. To test lymphocyte function in the laboratory, mitogen- and antigen-induced lymphocyte proliferation or transformation studies are performed. For these studies, lymphocytes are stimulated to proliferate involving new DNA synthesis and cell division. Lymphocytes from immunized or previously exposed individuals will normally proliferate in response to antigens to which they are sensitized, such as tetanus toxoid. This response *in vitro* correlates with the *in vivo* delayed-type

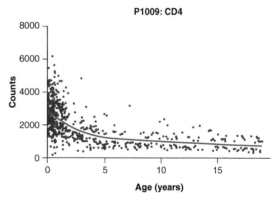

FIG. 6.3 Change in Distribution of Peripheral Blood CD4 T-Cell Subsets With Age in Healthy Children. Scatter plot indicates peripheral blood CD4 T-cell counts (cells/µL) by age, with lowest curves in healthy children from birth to 18 years of age. (From Shearer WT, et al. Lymphocyte subsets in healthy children from birth through 18 years of age: The Pediatric AIDS Clinical Trials Group P1009 study. J Allergy Clin Immunol 2003; 112: 973, with permission from Elsevier.)

hypersensitivity (DTH) DTH response. Mitogens, such as concanavalin A (ConA), phytohemagglutinin (PHA), and pokeweed mitogen (PWM), stimulate proliferation of normal T cells, as can allogeneic histocompatibility antigens when leukocytes from two donors are mixed in culture. Proliferation of lymphocytes can be evaluated by the demonstration of cell division or by increased DNA synthesis reflecting this cell process. Increased DNA synthesis is monitored by the incorporation of radiolabeled nucleotides, usually tritiated thymidine, in culture media. A measure of the amount of radioactivity in the cells correlates with DNA synthesis. Other assays to assess mitogen-induced cell proliferation measure deoxybromouridine incorporation, change in pH, or adenosine triphosphate (ATP) concentration of the culture media. These assays are being increasingly used as surrogate markers of cellular immunity; however, a comparison with the traditional assay based on radiolabeled nucleotide is not available. Of note, a flow cytometry assay that measures cell division with the use of carboxyl fluorescein succinyl ester (CFSE), a fluorescent compound that distributes evenly in cells and specific antibodies, is also increasingly used in clinical immunology.[11] CFSE is distributed equally in dividing cells, and each progeny cell has half the fluorescence intensity of CFSE compared with the parent cell, providing the basis to identify these dividing cells. After mitogen or antigen stimulation, mononuclear cells can be stained with specifically labeled antibodies, allowing the identification of cell subsets that proliferate. Other functional testing available in selected clinical immunology centers includes apoptosis assays, activation-induced CD40 ligand expression, and STAT1 phosphorylation.

Phagocytes

The laboratory evaluation of a patient with a suspected phagocyte deficiency should always begin with a CBC. Neutropenia is the most frequently encountered disorder of the phagocyte system.[12] Neutrophilia, at values exceeding those associated with acute infection, is a common finding in LAD type 1 (LAD-1). Abnormalities of WBC function involve difficulty with adherence, locomotion, deformability, recognition, attachment, engulfment, phagosome formation, phagocytosis, degranulation, microbial killing, and elimination of engulfed material. Clinical assays to evaluate neutrophil function are limited in number. Chronic granulomatous disease (CGD) is diagnosed by demonstrating absent or markedly reduced oxidase activity in neutrophils in response to stimulation. Oxidase activity can be

detected by a flow cytometry assay measuring the oxidation of dihydrorhodamine (DHR) 123 in phagocytes, resulting in fluorescent rhodamine-123.[13,14] The nitroblue tetrazolium (NBT) test measures oxidative burst activity as well, but it is a more subjective test and can miss the diagnosis of CGD. For patients with suspected LAD-1 deficiency, neutrophils are labeled with mAb directed against the adhesion molecule CD11/CD18 heterodimer. Absence of fluorescence intensity indicates lack of expression of the adhesion molecule. In addition, an increase of fluorescence intensity after stimulation can be documented in normal individuals, indicating the normal upregulation of this molecule after cell activation.[15] Other laboratory techniques used to identify phagocytic defects include assays for chemotaxis and bactericidal activity. A major pitfall for neutrophil studies is the spontaneous cell activation that might occur *in vitro* when cells are not tested within a few hours of when the sample was drawn, resulting in artifactual values that might falsely suggest poor function.

Complement

Laboratory tests for complement components include tests for functional activity of the classical pathway with a CH50 assay and the alternative pathway with an AH50 assay, as well as immunochemical methods to measure complement component levels.[16] The CH50 evaluation tests the ability of fresh serum from the patient to lyse antibody-coated sheep erythrocytes. This reflects the activity of all numbered components of the classical complement pathway, C1−C9, and terminal components of the alternative complement pathway. A total deficiency of one of the classical complement pathway components will result in a CH50 assay approaching zero. Patients with complement deficiency are rare, and complement test abnormalities are often transient because of increased consumption or activation due to an infection or an inflammatory condition. It is recommended that in case of an abnormal result, the complement test be repeated if the sample was taken when the patient had an acute illness. Quantitative tests for components C3 and C4 are utilized in testing for complement deficiencies and for evaluation of complement activation.

Innate Immunity: Interferon-γ Levels, Toll-Like Receptor Assay

The importance of the many components of innate immunity are increasingly recognized, as single gene defects in this immune compartment have been found to cause susceptibility to specific infections.[17,18] For example, patients with defects in the proteins that are part of the interferon-γ (IFN-γ) receptor may have elevated serum IFN-γ levels, even when there is no infection to explain these levels. The IFN-induced response associated kinase 4 (IRAK4) defect, observed with susceptibility to pneumococcal infection, might be accompanied with abnormal toll-like receptor (TLR) assay responses. The evaluation of NK-cell function and NK-cell phenotyping might be diagnostic for suspected familial hemophagocytic lymphohistiocytosis and other NK-cell deficiencies. It should be noted that the clinical value of most of these innate immunity tests as screening or diagnostic tools for immune defects has not been clearly established.

Many patients with increased frequency of infections may not have abnormal results in clinically available immunological testing, even when every compartment of the immune system is evaluated. In these difficult cases, referral to tertiary care and research centers for investigation of rare diseases is recommended.

MOLECULAR TESTS FOR PRIMARY IMMUNODEFICIENCY

Molecular testing for specific PIDs is available through commercial and research laboratories.[19] These are helpful to identify affected patients, affected fetuses prenatally, and carriers of genetic mutations. Biochemical and genetic testing should be considered. If autosomal recessive SCID is suspected, the adenosine deaminase (ADA) and purine nucleoside phosphorylase (PNP) enzyme activities in the RBCs should be determined. White blood cells must be used to measure the activity of these enzymes in recently transfused individuals, since donor RBCs will elevate the enzyme activity in deficient patients. Patients with ataxia-telangiectasia (AT) are found with elevated alpha-fetoprotein (AFP) levels along with variable abnormalities in B- and T-cell function.

Nearly 300 defective genes and gene products have been identified to result in congenital immunodeficiency syndromes.[20] The diagnosis of primary immunodeficiencies can be confirmed with molecular genetic analysis (Chapters 1 and 7). For example, in a patient with arrest of B-cell development at the pre-B-cell stage and agammaglobulinemia, gene testing might identify mutations in *BTK* leading to the absence of Bruton tyrosine kinase (BTK). Similarly, when there is evidence of abnormal T-cell development leading to SCID, gene testing might be able to identify deleterious mutations in 1 of 15 genes, including *IL2RG* and *JAK3*. In addition to gene sequencing, the study of copy number variation (CNV) by microarray assays or

karyotyping identify gene deletions or duplications that might explain the clinical presentation. Patients with possibly deleterious gene mutations that have not been investigated need to be carefully evaluated to demonstrate the pathogenic nature of the genetic change. Some genetic changes do not have clinical significance and are known as single nucleotide polymorphisms (SNPs). Standard protocols using Southern, Northern, and Western blot analyses, PCR analysis, and DNA sequence analysis are helpful to identify affected patients, affected fetuses prenatally, and carriers of genetic mutations. Most recently, the use of whole-exome sequencing for immunodeficiency syndromes has facilitated the identification of new genes causing immunodeficiencies by examining all known gene exons without bias.[21] This methodology for diagnosis is particularly helpful when the clinical presentation does not match any of the already described immunodeficiency syndromes.[22]

CONCLUSIONS

> **Clinical Pearls**
> *Laboratory Diagnosis of Immunodeficiency Patients*
>
> - Lymphopenia is a hallmark of T-cell immunodeficiency in infancy. Unexplained lymphopenia should be recognized and evaluated.
> - Normal range for immunoglobulin levels and lymphocyte counts varies with age; age-matched controls should be used for interpretation.
> - Implementation of universal screening of newborn infants by DNA analysis of dried blood spots on Guthrie cards (T-cell receptor excision circle [TREC]) detects all T-cell deficiencies.

The approach to the patient with suspected immune deficiency requires knowledge of developmental pathways and function of the different compartments of the immune system, as well as the clinical presentation of these disorders. The medical history, particularly the frequency, severity, and etiology of infections, is most helpful to orient the diagnostic workup. Commonly ordered tests in primary care, such as a CBC and serum Ig levels, are helpful to support possible diagnosis and referral to the clinical immunologist. Immunological testing according to clues obtained from the medical history helps narrow the differential diagnoses to specific immunodeficiencies, which are confirmed by molecular methods. Description of new T-cell subsets (*e.g.*, Th17 and regulatory T cells [Tregs]) has helped explain the immunopathogenesis of certain clinical manifestations, such as the occurrence of autoimmunity in patients with combined immunodeficiency, and "cold abscesses" in the autosomal dominant hyper-IgE syndrome (HIES). HIES. Testing for these lymphocyte phenotypes is being integrated in the clinical evaluation. Identification of genetic defects can now be accomplished by increased availability of whole-exome sequencing, as an alternative to genetic analysis of candidate genes. Technological advances are making molecular diagnosis available for most patients with immunodeficiency conditions.

> **On the Horizon**
>
> - Development of DNA sequence analysis for >350 types of primary immunodeficiency (PID).
> - Wide availability of whole-genome sequencing and chromosomal microarray methods to determine molecular defects for difficult to diagnose immunodeficiency syndromes.

REFERENCES

1. Yel L. Selective IgA deficiency. *J Clin Immunol*. 2010;30: 10−16.
2. Kwan A, Abraham RS, Currier R, et al. Newborn screening for severe combined immunodeficiency in 11 screening programs in the United States. *JAMA*. 2014;312:729−738.
3. Boyle JM, Buckley RH. Population prevalence of diagnosed primary immunodeficiency diseases in the United States. *J Clin Immunol*. 2007;27:497−502.
4. Shillitoe B, Bangs C, Guzman D, et al. The United Kingdom Primary Immune Deficiency (UKPID) registry 2012 to 2017. *Clin Exp Immunol*. 2018;192:284−291.
5. UNAIDS. AIDS by the numbers 2015. *Joint United Nations Programme on HIV/AIDS (UNAIDS) and World Health Organization (WHO)*. 2015.
6. Agarwal S, Mayer L. Diagnosis and treatment of gastrointestinal disorders in patients with primary immunodeficiency. *Clin Gastroenterol Hepatol*. 2013;11: 1050−1063.
7. Ozen A, Baris S, Karakoc-Aydiner E, et al. Outcome of hypogammaglobulinemia in children: immunoglobulin levels as predictors. *Clin Immunol*. 2010;137:374−383.
8. Balloch A, Licciardi PV, Russell FM, et al. Infants aged 12 months can mount adequate serotype-specific IgG responses to pneumococcal polysaccharide vaccine. *J Allergy Clin Immunol*. 2010;126:395−397.
9. Orange JS, Ballow M, Stiehm ER, et al. Use and interpretation of diagnostic vaccination in primary immunodeficiency: a working group report of the basic and clinical immunology interest section of the American Academy of Allergy Asthma & Immunology. *J Allergy Clin Immunol*. 2012;130:S1−24.
10. Johnson HL, Deloria-Knoll M, Levine OS, et al. Systematic evaluation of serotypes causing invasive pneumococcal disease among children under five: the pneumococcal global serotype project. *PLoS Med*. 2010;7:pii:e1000348.
11. Rakha A, Todeschini M, Casiraghi F. Assessment of anti-donor T cell proliferation and cytotoxic T lymphocyte-mediated lympholysis in living donor kidney transplant patients. *Methods Mol Biol*. 2014;1213:355−364.
12. Henry M, Sung L. Supportive care in pediatric oncology: oncologic emergencies and management of fever and neutropenia. *Pediatr Clin North Am*. 2015;62:27−46.
13. Holland SM. Chronic granulomatous disease. *Hematol Oncol Clin North Am*. 2013;27:89−99.
14. Yu JE, Chang HJ, Jongo AM, et al. Considerations in the diagnosis of chronic granulomatous disease. *J Pediatric Infect Dis Soc*. 2018;9(suppl 1):S6−S11.
15. Etzioni A. Defects in the leukocyte adhesion cascade. *Clin Rev Allergy Immunol*. 2010;38:54−60.
16. Grumach AS, Kirschfink M. Are complement deficiencies really rare? Overview on prevalence, clinical importance and modern diagnostic approach. *Mol Immunol*. 2014;61: 110−117.
17. Rosenzweig SD, Holland SM. Recent insights into the pathobiology of innate immune deficiencies. *Curr Allergy Asthma Rep*. 2011;11:369−377.
18. Bustamonte J, Zhang S-Y, Boisson B, et al. Immunodeficiencies at the interface of innate and adaptive immunity. In: Rich RR, et al., eds. *Clinical Immunology: Principles and Practice*. 5th ed. Elsevier; 2019:509.
19. https://www.genetests.org/tests/.
20. Picard C, Al-Herz W, Bousfiha A, et al. Primary immunodeficiency diseases: an update on the classification from the International Union of Immunological Societies expert committee for primary immunodeficiency 2015. *J Clin Immunol*. 2015;35:696−726.
21. Stray-Pedersen A, Sorte HS, Samarakoon P, et al. Primary immunodeficiency diseases: Genomic approaches delineate heterogeneous Mendelian disorders. *J Allergy Clin Immunol*. 2017;139:232−245.
22. Platt C, Geha RS, Chou J. Gene hunting in the genomic era: approaches to diagnostic dilemmas in patients with primary immunodeficiencies. *J Allergy Clin Immunol*. 2014; 134:262−268.

CHAPTER 7

Techniques in Genome Analysis

JOHN W. BELMONT

Molecular analysis of genes and genomes can be central to arriving at a precision diagnosis. This chapter reviews the basic principles that underlie clinical molecular genetic testing, assesses representative standard methods that are widely employed, describes new DNA sequencing methods that are being rapidly introduced into clinical diagnostic laboratories, and suggests a multidisciplinary approach for implementation in immunological disorders.

FUNDAMENTAL PRINCIPLES
Genome Structure and Gene Expression

> **Key Concepts**
> *Human Genomics*
>
> - The human genome encompasses approximately 20 000 protein-coding genes, but each cell expresses only a subset of those genes.
> - Genetic and physical maps of the genome are essential to molecular diagnosis of immune system diseases.
> - Genetic maps depend on the coinheritance of DNA segments—linkage—to associate DNA variants with disease.
> - Physical maps of the genome describe the exact gene locations on a chromosome. The genome DNA sequence is the finest scale physical map of the genome.

The human genome is thought to have about 20 000 protein-coding genes distributed on 23 pairs of chromosomes (http://www.ncbi.nlm.nih.gov/entrez/). The total length of one copy of the genome is $\approx 3 \times 10^9$ nucleotide bases. The protein-coding segments (exons) are split by noncoding DNA sequences (introns). The aggregate protein-coding sequences, referred to as the "exome," account for about 1–1.5% of the genome. Some of the remaining DNA contains regulatory elements that direct the expression of genes, control chromatin conformation, encode regulatory RNAs, act as origins for DNA replication, and participate in three-dimensional (3D) looping to produce the large-scale chromosome structure. About 40% of the total DNA is accounted for by families of repeated sequences. These repeat elements are generally silent, but they may be involved in some types of gene regulation and can become involved in mutational mechanisms of deletion, duplication, and insertion. Each cell expresses only a subset of the entire gene repertoire. "Housekeeping" genes are expressed in almost all tissues and cell types, where they perform basic metabolic and structural functions. Other genes are under very specific control, and their expression is restricted to one or a few cell types. Differential gene expression specifies the unique functions of cells (*e.g.*, immunoglobulin [Ig] in B cells, and T-cell receptor [TCR] in T cells). Genes that coordinate the expression of groups of tissue-specific genes primarily encode transcription factors that regulate the rate of messenger RNA (mRNA) transcription on their target genes. A few of these apparently act as "master" genes during particular developmental processes or in specific cell lineages. Some of these master genes (*e.g., PAX5*) may be involved in leukemias and lymphomas. So far, immunodeficiency genes appear to be in the category of genes that involve either innate or adaptive immunity controlling cell growth, differentiation, effector functions, or apoptosis.[1,2]

Polymorphic Variation and Linkage

A genetic map relates one gene to another based on how often they are inherited together. Within a specific region of the DNA, the maternal and paternal copies of the genome may be nonidentical, and the variants are called *alleles*. Protein and nucleotide differences are called *polymorphisms* when they are frequent enough to be found in 1–5% of the general population. Variations in single nucleotides occur in $\approx 1/100$ bases when whole-genome sequencing is used to survey individuals.[3] Polymorphisms arise over time in a group

Core Laboratory Technologies in Clinical Immunology. https://doi.org/10.1016/B978-0-323-66149-2.00007-4

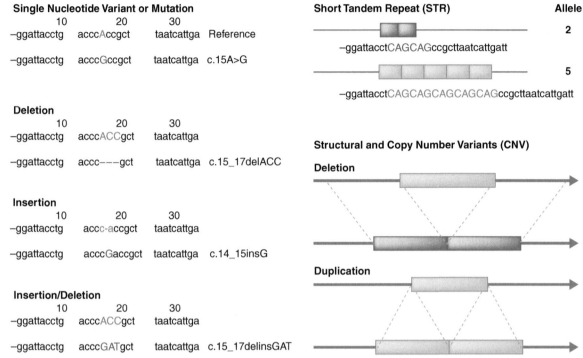

FIG. 7.1 Classes of DNA Variation Important for Genetic Testing and Human Genetic Diseases. DNA variations can be either benign or pathogenic, depending on whether they affect the underlying functions of a genetic locus and the encoded proteins. An international standard nomenclature is used to describe changes in the DNA. Structural variants have been found to be a common cause of human genetic disorders.

of individuals because of mutations in the DNA (Fig. 7.1). Some polymorphisms involve simple sequence repeats so that there is variation in the number of repeat units. These are called *short tandem repeats* (STRs) and are widely used in forensic identification. In contrast to STRs, the most common polymorphisms involve a change in a single nucleotide position. Large databases of single nucleotide polymorphisms (SNPs, pronounced "snips") have been accumulated (http://www.ncbi.nlm.nih.gov/SNP/). It is thought that there could be $>30 \times 10^6$ SNPs with minor allele frequency $>5\%$ available across the human genome. Many SNPs are found in noncoding DNA, and these have been shown to play a significant, albeit incompletely understood, role in common human diseases.

The composition of alleles within genetic loci in an individual is called the *genotype*. The individual's genotype interacts with the environment throughout life to create the *phenotype*. Some components of the phenotype, such as body weight, are simple to measure, whereas other clinically important phenotypes are based on complex laboratory evaluation

(*e.g.*, in T-cell proliferation). A key distinction is drawn between discrete traits (normal vs. abnormal) and quantitative traits (continuous range of values). Polymorphisms account for some of the variations observed at the phenotype level between healthy individuals or between populations, and the cumulative percentage of the variation explained by genetic variation is called *heritability*. In monogenic diseases (also called *mendelian diseases*), the presence of mutation(s) is usually considered necessary and sufficient to cause disease. The landscape of genetic variation in each individual includes a continuum of gene effects ranging from weak (common SNPs detected in disease association studies) to strongly determinative (rare mutations detected in single-gene disorders).

Genes can be mapped in relation to one another by a *linkage* map. Genes that are physically close can be shown to be predominantly coinherited. Linkage mapping played a large role in the identification of the X-linked immunodeficiency genes. Beyond small families and at the population level, the correlation of alleles among markers that are very close to each other in the genome is called *linkage disequilibrium* (LD). LD occurs because the mutation that creates a polymorphism occurs on a single chromosome with its whole complement of unique variants. This initial arrangement of alleles, however, is broken up by recombination over time. Hence, only markers that are relatively close to each other continue to have significant LD. A large international project (HapMap) created a dense map of SNP markers allowing a comprehensive view of LD in several reference populations.[4] This information has been efficiently exploited in genetic epidemiology projects called *genome-wide association studies* (GWAS; www.gwascentral.org), which have characterized several thousand common variants that contribute to many common immunological diseases, such as diabetes, rheumatoid arthritis (RA), and systemic lupus erythematosus (SLE).

The advent of projects that assess whole exomes and genomes in normal and disease populations, such as the 1000 Genomes Project (www.1000genomes.org/), has focused much more attention on rare genetic variation, particularly alleles with frequency of 0.01–1.0%. It is also apparent that the extent of individual genetic variation was underestimated from previous data and that each individual bears about 3.5 million simple nucleotide variants and about 1000 structural variants, many of which are unique to that person. Even given some technical reservations, the enormous extent of private variation has been clearly established.

Linkage and LD mapping have been much less useful for the identification of autosomal recessive genes responsible for many primary immunodeficiencies (PIDs) because the diseases are rare in the population and average families are not large enough to narrowly localize the causative genes. Whole-genome and whole-exome sequencing technologies are being used to solve a great fraction of remaining single-gene disorders, including PIDs.[5,6] The biggest difficulty with these conditions is that similar clinical diseases can be caused by mutation in more than one gene locus (*locus heterogeneity*). Another challenge is that it may be difficult to ascertain multiple extremely rare families with mutations in the same gene. Criteria for rare disease gene identification have been proposed and have helped harmonize standards for future genome interpretation.[7] Successful identification of pathogenic variants, even those unique to single pedigrees, can be accomplished by combining DNA sequencing with complimentary functional technologies.

Physical Maps and DNA Copy Number Variation

Physical maps are different from the genetic map in that they describe how genes are arranged in the DNA on a scale as large as a whole chromosome and as fine as a single nucleotide. At the coarsest level of the physical map, genes are placed in chromosome segments corresponding to the Giemsa-stain banding pattern of metaphase chromosomes. A way to localize genes is to hybridize region-specific DNA probes directly to a chromosome spread. The technique, called *fluorescence in situ hybridization* (FISH), allows the detection of signals from the chromosome spread to directly localize genes.[8] FISH is used for cytogenetic examination of tumors, leukemias, and lymphomas but now has been largely replaced by array *comparative genome hybridization* (CGH), which examines many hundreds of thousands of positions using oligonucleotide probes.[9] High-density oligonucleotide arrays allow for both standardization of reagents between diagnostic laboratories and extensive customization for particular disease applications. These methods are detailed below. Pathogenic *copy number variants* (CNVs) are a major cause of birth defects and intellectual disability,[10] so evaluation for CNVs should be considered a first-line test for any infant or child with a complex presentation of immune deficiency. In DiGeorge syndrome (DGS), the characteristic deletion of chromosome 22q11 can be detected by microarray. FISH should not be used because microarray not only provides high-resolution determination of the deletion size but also leaves open the possibility of detecting other unsuspected DNA copy number abnormalities.

Mutation and Pathogenic Variants

Key Concepts
Mutation

- Mutation can occur by deletion, insertion, or duplication of short or long DNA segments.
- Single-base mutations can be caused by replication errors or by chemical deamination of methylcytosine.
- Single-base mutations can affect protein-coding sequences, regulatory sequences, or the RNA splice signals within a gene.
- The parental origin of mutations (maternal or paternal) affects those mutational mechanisms most likely responsible.
- A disease can be caused by mutations in several alternative genes (locus heterogeneity).
- Most primary immunodeficiencies occur because of different kinds of mutations in particular genes (allelic heterogeneity).

DNA variants can involve single nucleotide substitutions, small or large deletions, insertions, inversions, duplications, or repeat expansions.[11] Some variants have no measurable or functionally significant phenotypic effect. They become one of the huge pool of neutral polymorphisms in the genome. Single-base substitutions in a triplet amino acid codon often disturb the normal function of proteins. These are described as *missense* (*i.e.*, causing an amino acid substitution) or *nonsense* (*i.e.*, terminating translation) mutations. Mutations affecting regulatory or splice signal sequences in RNA can also be deleterious. The primary mechanisms of mutation are misincorporation of nucleotides and faulty repair of chemically damaged nucleotides (*e.g.*, 8-oxodG) during DNA replication by DNA polymerases. Another important mechanism underlying single base or "point" mutations occurs at CpG dinucleotides. The cytosine is often methylated, and chemical deamination of the methylated cytosine gives the base thymidine. At the next round of replication the CG may be changed to TG or CA, depending on which DNA strand was altered. Small insertion and deletion (*indel*) mutations are also very common. Indels occurring in protein-coding sequence are usually deleterious, as they can cause frameshifts (changing the reading frame, leading to translation termination within a few codons) and account for almost 25% of known human disease-causing mutations.[12] They result from strand slippage in repetitive sequences and misaligned intermediates during DNA synthesis. An entirely different mechanism for mutation is expansion of short repeat segments (most often trinucleotides).[13] So far, no disorder that affects the immune system has been associated with this mechanism.

Heritable mutations can arise in either the male or the female germline, but the gender-related frequency is influenced by the mutational mechanism. Chromosomal nondisjunction, for example, occurs predominantly during female meiosis and has a strong maternal age effect.[14,15] The fact that spermatogonial proliferation occurs throughout life and involves many more cell replications than oogenesis increases the single-base mutation frequency in the paternal germline.[16,17] Clinicians must cope with both locus and allele heterogeneity. *Locus heterogeneity* means that the same or a similar phenotype results from mutation in one of several different genes. For example, severe combined immunodeficiency (SCID) can result from mutation in the adenosine deaminase, interleukin-2 (IL-2) receptor γ-chain genes, *JAK3*, and so on. *Allelic heterogeneity* means that the disease is caused by different mutations in the same gene. In X-linked disorders, allelic heterogeneity is typically high because affected individuals have reduced reproduction (negative evolutionary selection), and most mutations are lost in the population after a few generations. At autosomal loci, some mutations have reached appreciable frequency as a result of demographic processes (*e.g.*, *founder effect*). In the heterozygous state, recessive mutations can be weakly deleterious, neutral, or actually confer a small advantage. Because the mutant alleles are common, it is possible to test affected individuals and potential carriers directly for those mutations. This is the basis for population screening for carrier status in cystic fibrosis. However, none of the immune deficiencies results from common mutations that would permit efficient screening. In the autosomal recessive immune deficiencies, most patients have two different, very rare mutations (*compound heterozygosity*) at the disease locus. If there is known parental consanguinity or the family comes from an isolated population, the affected individual may be homozygous for a rare mutation.

X-Chromosome Inactivation

Disturbances in the pattern of X inactivation are interesting phenomena in women who are carriers of X-linked disorders, including several immune deficiencies.[18] Measurement of X-chromosome activity in the blood cells of normal women shows that, on average, the contribution of maternal and paternal X chromosomes is approximately 50 : 50. Extreme skewing of X inactivation often results from abnormal proliferation of blood cells. X-inactivation analysis can be used to demonstrate clonal growth of premalignant (*e.g.*, myelodysplasia) and malignant cells. In a female carrying mutations at the X-linked severe combined immune deficiency (*XSCID*; OMIM 300400), agammaglobulinemia (*XLA*; OMIM 300300), or Wiskott-Aldrich syndrome (*WAS*; OMIM 301000) loci, cell competition and compensation mechanisms lead to a reduced contribution of cells expressing the mutant allele among affected cells. In XLA, the B-cell lineage shows selective use of the nonmutant active X chromosome. In XSCID, skewing of X inactivation is observed in B cells, T cells, and natural killer (NK) cells. In WAS, some degree of skewing of X inactivation results from defective hematopoietic stem cell (HSC) activity. Historically, skewed X inactivation was very helpful in linkage mapping of these conditions. As a clinical test, X inactivation now has reduced importance compared with direct mutation analyses.

PRINCIPLES AND DESCRIPTION OF DNA DIAGNOSTIC TECHNIQUES

The overriding theme of all DNA diagnostic techniques is the detection of variants in the DNA molecule that are associated with disease. This has historically involved a targeted search in one or a few specific genes or regions, but the field is evolving rapidly toward techniques that allow for simultaneous survey of the entire genome. DNA copy number analysis and DNA sequencing have come to dominate individual genetic diagnostic methods. Bioinformatics is a necessary diagnostic laboratory discipline that must be coupled to these methods, particularly when the whole genome is surveyed.

Detection of Disease-Causing Copy Number Variants: FISH and Microarrays

Many genetic diseases are caused by deletions or duplications in human DNA. These conditions typically have copy number abnormalities ranging from 500 kilobases (Kb) to 5 megabases (Mb) and are sometimes referred to as "genomic disorders." The most common genomic disorder with a clinically important effect on the immune system is 22q11 deletion syndrome. This disorder affects about 1 per 4000 live-born infants and accounts for about 90% of DGS cases. The karyotype, in which a metaphase chromosome spread was stained and visualized under the microscope, was for many decades the only clinically useful test for the detection of copy number changes. The karyotype offered a genome-wide view, but at a very low resolution; alterations smaller than 5 Mb, including those that typically cause DGS, were not routinely detected. Two methods, described below, have replaced conventional karyotypes for routine genetic diagnosis. Whole-genome sequencing (WGS) combined with advanced bioinformatics methods promises to transform evaluation of CNVs yet again. In principle, the data collected in WGS can be used to resolve all CNVs regardless of length, thus capturing all forms of structural DNA variation from the smallest to gross abnormalities in chromosomes.

Fluorescence *In Situ* Hybridization

FISH has been an important technology for detecting both constitutional and somatic abnormalities in chromosomes.[19] In its simplest form, a cloned gene segment (referred to as a *probe*) is labeled (Fig. 7.2)

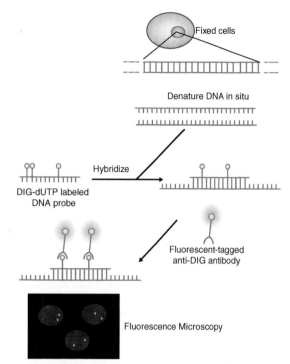

FIG. 7.2 Fluorescence *in situ* Hybridization (FISH). Probes complementary to specific sites in the genome are labeled with a hapten (*e.g.*, digoxigenin) and then hybridized to denatured DNA within cells on microscope slides. The hybridized probes are then detected by immunofluorescence microscopy.

and allowed to hybridize to a preparation of early metaphase (condensed) chromosomes. The labeled probe hybridizes specifically to a locus and is then detected with secondary antibodies and high-sensitivity immunofluorescence techniques. The targeted locus appears as two pairs of dots corresponding to the sister chromatids from the two chromosomal homologues. Cells that are in interphase (when the DNA is largely unfolded in the nucleus) can also be probed. In the interphase cell, two single signals are observed corresponding to the two chromosomes. With the introduction of microarray-based methods for genome-wide copy number analysis, the practical application of FISH has been narrowed but does have a continuing role in defining balanced translocations and in cancer cytogenetics.

Array-Based Copy Number Analysis

> ### Key Concepts
> #### Molecular Methods
>
> - Most DNA diagnostics rely on DNA copy number analysis or DNA sequencing.
> - Polymerase chain reaction (PCR) allows for exponential amplification of a DNA segment from the genome, allowing multiple analytical procedures on the single pure sequence.
> - Array-based copy number analysis has become the first-line method for finding small abnormalities in the structure of chromosomes.
> - New high-throughput sequencing methods have emerged as practical alternatives to older single analysis approaches.
> - Bioinformatics is an emerging discipline relevant to molecular diagnosis. Integration of bioinformatics techniques plays a necessary role in data acquisition and interpretation.

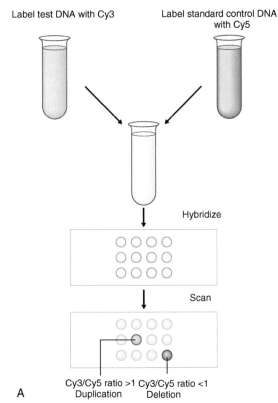

Oligonucleotide arrays have had a revolutionary impact on molecular diagnostics, by offering high-resolution, genome-wide detection of copy number changes. The basic principle involves synthetic oligonucleotides complementary to human nucleic acid sequences bound to a surface or bead, and hybridization of fragmented, labeled human nucleic acid samples (Fig. 7.3). Array printing of activated phosphoramidite nucleotide precursors allows for hundreds to thousands of oligonucleotides to be fabricated on activated glass surfaces (Agilent Technologies, Santa Clara, CA).[20] Light-activated oligonucleotide synthesis has also been used to efficiently customize oligonucleotide arrays (Affymetrix Inc., Santa Clara, CA; and Roche Nimblegen Inc., Madison, WI).[21] A third approach involves synthesis of oligonucleotides on microbeads that are randomly flowed over a patterned surface (Illumina Inc., San Diego, CA).[22,23] These processes are very similar, in principle, to the fabrication of microelectronic devices and so have given these arrays the nickname "gene chips."

Microarrays have been used in very-large-scale studies to genotype common polymorphisms. Robust chemistries that can analyze standard sets of up to 5 000 000 SNPs in a single assay are now routine (see Fig. 7.3). Nonamplified genomic DNA is too complex (*i.e.*, the concentration of any particular sequence is too low) to be analyzed directly. High-throughput genotyping assays require an array-

FIG. 7.3 Array-Based DNA Copy Number Analysis. (A) Array comparative genomic hybridization (aCGH) uses a reference DNA to compare with the test DNA. The labeled DNA is hybridized to an array of oligonucleotides that are designed to be uniquely complementary to hundreds of thousands of positions in the genome. The relative intensities of the fluorescence signal from each DNA probe allow assessment of copy number. Cy3 and Cy5 are cyanine conjugated fluorescent dyes. Genotyping arrays are also widely used for copy number testing (B and C). (B) Whole-genome sampling and amplification (WGSA). End-labeled polymerase chain reaction (PCR) products that constitute a sample from the genome are hybridized to oligo sets on standard chips. The oligos are organized into "probe quartets" consisting of perfect matches (PMs) and single-base mismatches (MMs) for each allele (A and B). Separate quartets for the sense and antisense strand of DNA help to ensure specificity, and in the actual assay these quartets are repeated three to five times on the chip. This type of assay has been developed to test a standard panel of >2 million DNA features per sample. (C) Single-base extension (SBE; Illumina Infinium II). This assay uses whole-genome amplification (WGA) to increase the molar concentration of target DNA. SBE on arrays of tagged microbeads allows allele discrimination, and the resulting products are detected by immunostaining (signal amplification). This assay has been used for assays of up to 5 million single nucleotide polymorphisms (SNPs) per sample.

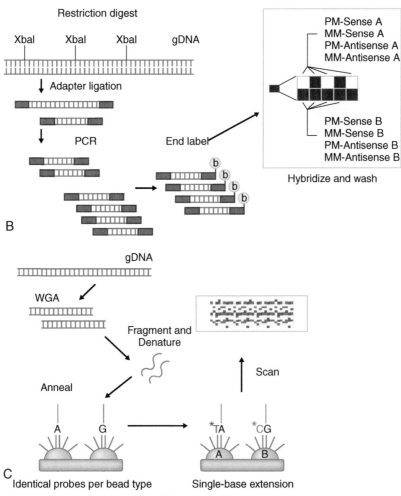

FIG. 7.3, cont'd.

based readout and scalable, multiplex assay chemistry. This is extremely challenging because of the complexity of the human genome (*i.e.,* any particular unique sequence in the mixture has a low molar concentration) and because of the need for exquisite specificity at the single-base level. An important general principle for achieving single-base specificity is the detection of physically coincident events.[24] This is exactly the route taken by the polymerase chain reaction (PCR), in which specific annealing of both primers is required for the reaction to take place (Fig. 7.4).

Whole-genome sampling and amplification (WGSA) implemented in the Affymetrix SNP arrays uses parallel amplification of short DNA segments (200–1100 base pairs [bp]) that are then labeled and hybridized to oligonucleotide probe arrays.[25] The oligonucleotides are specific for each allele of SNPs, and the resulting hybridization intensities can be used to derive the genotypes. These assays are fixed in the sense that the investigator uses the information from a standardized array but cannot add SNPs for particular purposes. An alternative approach, incorporated in the Infinium assays (Illumina Inc., San Diego, CA), involves the detection of allele-specific primer extension or single-base extension products on a self-assembling high-density microbead array.[26] In the Infinium assays, genomic DNA is first subjected to whole-genome amplification (WGA), and those products are hybridized to an array of locus-specific 50-mer capture probes. Either primer extension or ligation reactions on the array surface are used to accomplish allele discrimination. Signal amplification with methods familiar to users of enzyme-linked immunosorbent assay (ELISA) is used to enhance the sensitivity. A distinct advantage of this class

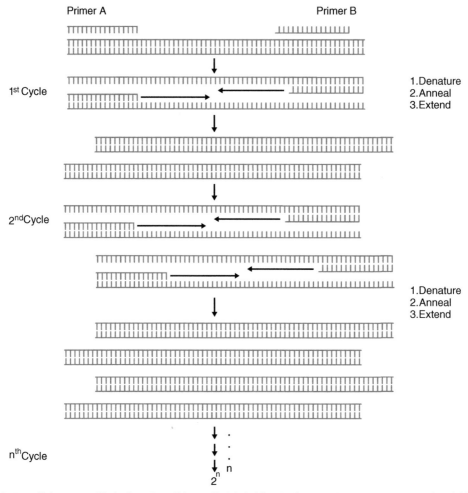

FIG. 7.4 Polymerase Chain Reaction. Primers that hybridize to the target sequence are used to initiate multiple cycles of synthesis, melting, annealing, and synthesis. In practice, the potential geometrical increase in DNA tapers off as reaction components become limiting.

of assays is that the "assay conversion" (percent SNPs that actually allow inference of the genotype in the final assay mixture) is very high and thus allows for flexibility in designing tests customized to particular problems.

GENE EXPRESSION

Global gene expression analysis has been enabled by microarray technology giving rise to so-called "transcriptomics." For RNA expression analysis, cDNA "target" derived from the tissue or cell source is labeled with fluorophores and used to determine complementary binding by massively parallel hybridization to the probes fixed on the array. The ability to massively sequence RNA (see below) from

diverse biological samples has reduced use of arrays for research. RNA measurement, either by array or sequencing, has been slow to enter clinical practice. A major challenge lies in the variation between studies in sample selection, cell composition of samples, analysis platform, and statistical methods. Establishing criteria for analytical validity, clinical validity, and clinical utility are long-term challenges for use of gene expression biomarkers.

Detection of Disease-Causing Mutations—Point Mutations, Insertions/ Deletions, and Structural Variants

Methods for the detection of single-base substitutions in DNA are central to clinical genetic diagnostics.[27]

Although complementary DNA (cDNA) synthesized from mRNA can be used, analysis of genomic DNA is far more common. Many different methods for mutation detection have been described, but virtually all clinical diagnostic laboratories now approach an unknown mutation with DNA sequencing. When Sanger sequencing is used, the first step is to design PCR primer sets that will allow amplification of each exon. The availability of the reference human genome sequence makes determination of gene structure and amplimer design for genomic DNA straightforward. Any mutation that directly affects amplification, such as deletion or mutation in the amplimer sequence, can produce misleading results. It is always desirable to have parental specimens available to serve as a reference for proving biallelic inheritance in the affected offspring. If there is a clear clinical diagnosis and only a single gene likely to be involved, then automated fluorescent sequencing is still the preferred method. For disorders with highly complex clinical and laboratory phenotypes, like primary immune deficiencies, the problem of locus heterogeneity is very severe. It is now routine practice to solve this problem by sequencing the complete exome or the complete genome in individual patients by using the next-generation technologies described below.

Sanger Sequencing

The direct determination of a DNA sequence is fundamental to mutation identification (Fig. 7.5). The oldest method still in common use (called *Sanger sequencing*) depends on termination of DNA synthesis by chemically modified nucleotides (dideoxynucleotide triphosphates [ddNTPs]). A single-stranded DNA (ssDNA) template is hybridized to a primer that can recognize a short known segment of DNA. The ssDNA is usually produced by DNA amplification. The primer acts as a starting point for DNA synthesis by a DNA polymerase that is added to the reaction. Four separate reactions are set up, each "spiked" with one of the four possible ddNTPs (ddATP, ddTTP, ddCTP, or ddGTP). As synthesis proceeds, some of the strands incorporate a ddNTP, and no further extension can take place. In each reaction, a family of molecules is synthesized; their unit lengths are determined by whether the reaction had been terminated by incorporation of a specific ddNTP at a given position. Either the primer or the nucleotides may be labeled. Automated instrumentation for DNA sequencing using laser scanning of fluorophore-labeled reactions is standard. By using four different fluorescent labels the reaction products from one sample can be analyzed together, with many samples processed in parallel using renewable capillary electrophoresis arrays.

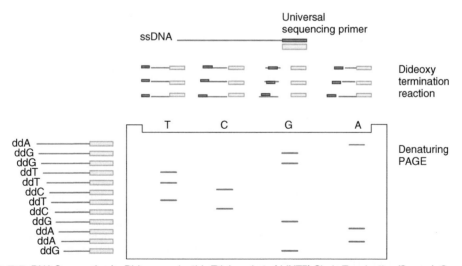

FIG. 7.5 DNA Sequencing by Dideoxynucleotide Triphosphate (ddNTP) Chain Termination (Sanger). Copying of the DNA by the polymerase is terminated at specific positions when a ddNTP is incorporated. The ddNTP is mixed with deoxynucleotide triphosphates (dNTPs) so that in each reaction, only some new strands terminate, whereas others continue through to the next complementary nucleotide. The sequencing products can be visualized by autoradiography or by laser scanning in an automated sequencer.

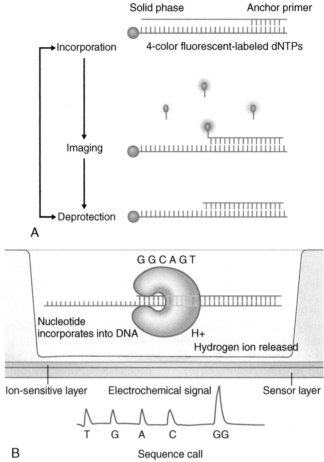

FIG. 7.6 Next-Generation DNA Sequencing. (A) Sequencing by synthesis (Illumina Inc., San Diego, CA). This is a method in which fluorescent-labeled terminator nucleotides are sequentially added and then imaged. After deprotection, another cycle of addition and imaging can take place. The currently available instrumentation allows simultaneous imaging of >1 billion "clusters" representing unique DNA elements. Approximately 100–150 cycles of base addition is commonly used. (B) Electrochemical sequencing (IonTorrent/ Proton; ThermoFisher Scientific, Waltham, MA). This method is very different from all others currently available in that it does not use any fluorescence labels or imaging. Sequences are inferred by changes in electrical conductance caused by release of hydrogen ions when bases are added to a DNA chain. (C) Single-molecule sequencing (PacBio, Pacific Biosciences, Menlo Park, CA). In this method DNA polymerase is attached in a microscope imaging unit called a zero-mode waveguide (ZMW). A single DNA molecule is imaged as fluorescent nucleotides are added on the single-stranded template DNA. This method distinguishes itself by the very rapid rate of reaction and the very long read length achieved. (D) Nanopore sequencing uses protein nanopores arrayed in a membrane. DNA passing through the pore causes a slight disruption in the current making it possible to identify the base at each position in the sequence. Oligonucleotides and motor enzymes tethers are used to attach the DNA to the pore and cause the DNA to move through the pore, respectively.

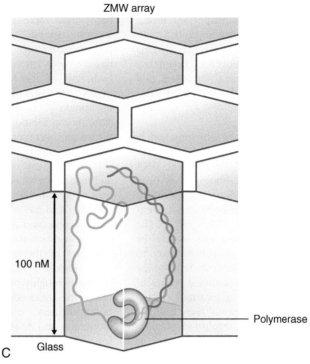

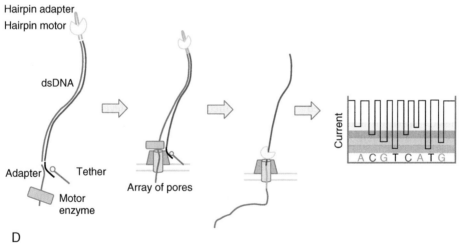

FIG. 7.6, cont'd.

Next-Generation DNA Sequencing

New technologies that have dramatically increased the throughput and reduced the cost of DNA sequencing have been rapidly adopted in research and diagnostic laboratories. Unlike Sanger sequencing, which produces sequence data by controlled termination of the polymerase, the new techniques derive the sequence as nucleotides are sequentially added by the polymerase or interrogate the sequence by flow through nanopores. Although multiple chemistries and detection systems have been developed into sequencing instruments (Fig. 7.6), this discussion will review methods that have been adopted into clinically validated assays and also briefly describe two methods that, to date, have only been used in research but that illustrate the potential for very long reads. Such methods may have a role in better defining structural variants in DNA. In addition, an important recent application of next-generation sequencing (NGS) will be discussed, circulating cell-free DNA (cfDNA). This technology has already revolutionized pregnancy screening for common chromosomal disorders and may be adapted to screening for low levels of solid tumor DNA in blood.

Sequencing by synthesis (Illumina). The most widely used system for NGS involves highly parallel imaging of single-base addition on "clusters" of identical DNA molecules (see Fig. 7.6A). This technology has been commercialized by Illumina Inc. (San Diego, CA). In their approach, DNA is ligated to primers that allow it to be amplified on a surface called a "flow cell."[28] The DNA templates attach to the flow cell surface by hybridization to specific primers complementary to that used to prepare the DNA library. Solid-phase bridge amplification creates many identical copies of each single template molecule in a localized cluster. The density of the clusters is extremely high, and the specialized imaging system allows resolution of more than 10^9 clusters per flow cell. DNA sequence is determined in the flow cell by sequential addition of fluorescent-tagged nucleotides. A single-labeled nucleotide is added to nascent DNA in each sequencing cycle. Each nucleotide has a different fluorophore so that all four are added to the mix in each cycle of base extension. The nucleotide label also terminates polymerization (*i.e.*, only a single base is added at each cycle), and the identity of the incorporated nucleotide is determined by the fluorescent emission spectrum and intensity. Because the bases act as terminators, homopolymeric segments can be resolved relatively accurately. After each deoxynucleotide triphosphate (dNTP) incorporation, the fluorescent dye is enzymatically cleaved to allow incorporation of the next nucleotide. This class of instruments is capable of sequencing complete human genomes in a single run.

Electrochemical sequencing. Electrochemical sequencing (IonTorrent/Proton; ThermoFisher Scientific, Waltham, MA) is distinctly different from systems that image fluorescent-tagged nucleotides because the sensor is a microelectronic device (see Fig. 7.6B).[29] DNA is first fragmented and then ligated to adapters, and the adapter-ligated libraries are clonally amplified by emulsion PCR onto beads. Individual beads are then loaded into single-sensor wells. Nucleotides are provided in a stepwise fashion with incorporation

increasing the length of the sequencing primer by one base when there is a complementary base on the template strand. Sequence determination relies on primer extension. Nucleotide incorporation into a nascent DNA strand by DNA polymerase results in hydrolysis of the nucleotide triphosphate. Hydrolysis causes production of a hydrogen ion for each nucleotide incorporated. The small shift in the pH of the surrounding solution is proportional to the number of nucleotides incorporated, which is then detected by the sensor on the bottom of each well, converted to a voltage, and digitized by off-chip electronics. The chip is automatically washed, and the cycle is repeated with the next nucleotide. Because of the small size of the wells, diffusion into and out of the well is very fast. The sensor layer is composed of tantalum oxide, which is sensitive to proton concentration (essentially pH) allowing rapid detection of the voltage transients that follow base incorporation in each well individually. The voltage change is roughly proportion to the length of a run of the same nucleotide in the DNA so that short homopolymers can be accurately called. Chip fabrication and design are very similar to methods used for microelectronic devices. This suggests that the method will have good potential to scale-up to increase the number of molecules processed in parallel. Lacking optical components, the cost of the all-electronic detection system is far less than other sequencing instruments.

Long read sequencing—single-molecule sequencing and nanopores. A true single-molecule sequencing method has been developed by Pacific Biosciences (Menlo Park, CA).[30] In their method DNA polymerase is immobilized in a femtoliter-sized well with special optical properties called the zero-mode waveguide (ZMW) (see Fig. 7.6C). The small size of the ZMW "hole" prevents 600-nm wavelength laser light from passing entirely through, and only the bottom 30 nm where the polymerase is bound is subject to the fluorescence excitation. Labeled nucleotides are flowed into the chamber, and complementary bases encountering the DNA polymerase are incorporated into the growing DNA chain. During incorporation, the DNA polymerase holds the nucleotide for tens of milliseconds, orders of magnitude longer than the average diffusing nucleotide. The transient light emission is then detected and the identity of the incorporated base recorded. Nucleotides with a fluorescent dye attached to the phosphate group of the nucleotide are cleaved when the nucleotide is incorporated into the DNA strand. The label diffuses away, leaving the DNA ready for the addition of the next base. The polymerase incorporates multiple bases per second, so the sequencing process is very fast with real-time observation of DNA synthesis.

Engineered nanopores are being evaluated for the detection of a broad array of biomolecules, including proteins and nucleic acids.[31] There are many potential variations in pore, sample preparation, and detection, which have given rise to active academic and commercial research programs. In one effective version, a protein channel (*e.g., Mycobacterium smegmatis* porin A, MspA) through which DNA may pass is held in a partition (membrane or other solid) that separates solutions containing charged ions. An applied voltage leading to movement of ions through the protein pore produces a measurable electrical current. DNA passing through the channel causes partial reduction of the current with the four DNA bases affecting the current by differing and characteristic amounts (see Fig. 7.6D). The changing electrical current is then used to infer the order of bases in the DNA molecule. Oxford Nanopore Technologies (Oxford, UK) released the first commercial devices based on this technology, and the uses are under active investigation. One of the most important strengths of this method is the very long single-molecule reads that can be obtained. High read depth can partially overcome problems with sequence accuracy (per base error rates of 10–30%). The fast run times and simple protocols for sample preparation have allowed an early stage instrument to be used to sequence Ebola virus on site in Africa. Because of the speed of analysis, "bedside" medical applications could be feasible (especially when base error rate is of less importance for the intended use) and appear especially promising in the arena of precision diagnosis of infectious diseases.

BIOINFORMATICS

Clinical Bioinformatics has emerged as a fundamental discipline in laboratory medicine, as enormous DNA sequence, transcriptomics, and variant databases have been aggregated from individual laboratories and international genomics projects. The growing number of genetic loci that are already known to be important in immunological disease renders it critical that diagnostic laboratories make maximal use of automated processes in sample management, data acquisition, data analysis, and reporting. Laboratories using NGS instruments must establish an informatics pipeline for each clinical application. New assay development requires validation conforming to Clinical Laboratory Improvement Amendments of 1988 (CLIA 1988) regulations, and laboratories must have an ongoing process to monitor data quality and ensure result accuracy. The US Food and Drug Administration (FDA) has released guidance on standards for clinical NGS-based diagnostic tests (https://www.fda.gov/downloads/MedicalDevices/DeviceRegulationandGuidance/GuidanceDocuments/UCM509838.pdf).

Sample and Laboratory Process Management

Each diagnostic laboratory must deal with the generic operational problems of sample accession, tracking, and reporting. Clinical-grade laboratory information management systems (LIMS) are required to handle all these processes with associated regulatory compliance. DNA diagnostic laboratories have several unique problems and requirements that deserve comment. Automated data acquisition is an important component of DNA sequencing and genotyping requiring personnel specialized in information science and systems administration. Advanced statistical models are employed at many steps in the processes of base calling (*primary analysis*), alignment to the reference genome, and identification of positions that are different from the reference (together called *secondary analysis*). Once the raw data from arrays and NGS are produced, bioinformaticians develop, manage, and operate analysis pipelines that synthesize the results into forms comprehensible to the laboratory staff tasked with reporting the results. Bioinformaticians maintain or develop analysis information management systems (AIMS), which are also used to collect and monitor performance metrics and quality control. Specialized software is used to perform these functions and to report the metrics needed for quality control. The number of patient-specific data records and the complexity of relationships in family-based testing make it essentially impossible for manual processes to achieve the required reliability. Because of the broad intended use of genomic testing, there is an increasing importance to collection of patient phenotype data, which is needed for variant filtering and prioritization (see Tertiary Data Analysis below).

Primary Data Analysis—Genotyping and Base Calling

Genotyping in the case of microarray and base calling in the case of sequencers are platform specific, and the required software is supplied by instrument vendors. Microarray data, whether array comparative genomic hybridization or SNP chip platforms, use signal hybridization intensity to estimate DNA copy number. Copy number calls are based on multiple adjacent assay positions with respect to the genome map (*i.e.*, the identification of clinically important CNVs is always supported by many independent data points and on-chip assay replicates). The resolution and reliability of the CNV calls depend on total number of positions on the array and their "responsiveness" to differences in DNA copy number. Laboratories using these methods must assess data quality with robust statistical procedures specifying in advance the minimum size and composition of so-called CNVs.

Sequencing data, especially when considering exome and whole genomes, presents much more challenging problems in bioinformatics. Base calling from the instrument raw data (primary analysis) typically takes place in local computers dedicated to the sequencer, but cloud-based methods can be used. Base calling generates sequence "reads" with their base quality scores. Some of the important measures of data quality at the primary analysis step are base quality score, number of reads per sample, length of reads, and fall-off of base quality with read position.

Secondary Data Analysis—Demultiplexing, Alignment, and Variant Calling

The next steps in next-generation sequence data analysis involve aligning reads to a reference sequence and generating variant calls. In many high-throughput applications, patient DNA samples are tagged with index sequences during preparation for sequencing (*library construction*). Molecular indexing or multiplexing allows pooling of the samples on the instrument and then sorting them out after sequencing. Demultiplexing of sequence reads is another step that is subject to quality monitoring.

After demultiplexing, the reads are mapped and aligned to the reference genome. Alignment of short-read sequences to the reference genome involves systematically matching read fragments to their correct location in the genome. The most widely used tools exploit the Burrow-Wheeler algorithm to carry out this process efficiently and precisely (bio-bwa.sourceforge.net/). Typically, only uniquely mapping reads are passed to the later steps of sequence analysis. This makes it difficult to analyze some segments of the genome that are important in health and disease. Some elements in the genome are composed of nearly identical sequences most often arranged in tandem on adjacent segments of chromosomes. Human leukocyte antigen (HLA) presents particular challenges: (*i*) certain HLA alleles may not be represented in the reference genomes; (*ii*) reads may align to more than one location in HLA leading to discard of the read or misalignment and false-positive variation; and (*iii*) identical reads may have origins in distinct haplotypes that cannot be easily recognized with short-read sequences.

Another important issue is that the reliability of variant calling is different with different classes of variation. Small insertion and deletion variants (indels) are clinically important because they often lead to frameshift and premature termination of proteins; but calling indels and automated application of consistent indel nomenclature are more difficult than single nucleotide variants (SNVs). The Genome Analysis Toolkit (http://www.broadinstitute.org/gatk/) is the most widely used software for variant calling.

Targeted resequencing and whole-exome sequencing (WES) focus on protein-coding elements in the genome. Because of the complex and highly variable exon-intron structure of genes, there is considerable technical difficulty in using exon sequence data to call structural variants and CNVs. WGS, in contrast, surveys all the intron and intergenic sequence. New methods of PCR-free library construction enable the read count depth to be used as an accurate surrogate for copy number.[32] In addition, gaps in aligned reads (called "split reads") can be used to recognize deletions and other structural variants, including duplications and inversions. Although challenges still remain, it is possible that WGS data combined with standardized algorithms could allow a single test to be used for almost all classes of pathogenic alleles.

Variants are saved in a specified format called a *genomic variant call format (gVCF) file*. This format contains information not only about the positions that contain a nonreference genotype call but also about the quality of each site that is called with the reference homozygous base. This is important because it allows multiple samples to be aggregated (*e.g.*, to analyze mother, father, and their offspring jointly). Format standardization allows exchange and aggregation of data among laboratories around the world. Data aggregation is now widely recognized as a key step in the development of molecular diagnostics, not only to reduce errors in variant calling but also to enable sophisticated approaches to the problem of genotype-phenotype relationships in rare genetic diseases.

Tertiary Data Analysis—Variant Annotation, Interpretation, and Reporting

The next steps in the analysis involve annotation, filtering, and classification of variants as to their likely role in the disease or phenotype for which the test was submitted. The laboratory must ensure that the final report is accurate and complete without overinterpretation. Annotation of each variant detected in the sequencing means attaching information about population frequency (or lack of previous observation), differences in frequency between various ethnic groups, effect of the variant on protein-coding sequence, effect on splicing, and so on. Diagnostic laboratories must actively use information contained in the public sequence databases to interpret the biological consequences of mutations and polymorphisms. There are databases that have an important role: *(i)* GenBank, which contains the reference human genome sequences (http://www.ncbi.nlm.nih.gov/entrez); *(ii)* dbSNP, which contains more than 150 000 000 common single nucleotide polymorphisms; *(iii)* Exome Sequencing Project (https://esp.gs.washington.edu/drupal/), which has exome data on about 6500 individuals from several research projects; *(iv)* the 1000 Genomes Project (http://www.1000genomes.org/), which has exome and genome data from about 2500 multiethnic controls; and *(v)* Exome Aggregation Consortium (http://exac.broadinstitute.org/), which has assembled variant data on more than 120 000 subjects from various diseases and population studies.

Interpretation of sequence and genotype information is the next step in carrying out a molecular diagnostic test. The laboratory must do the following: take into consideration the patient's presenting symptoms and other clinical data; examine the strength of the evidence that specific gene mutations can cause the suspected disease; look for variants in genes that might provide a causal explanation; determine whether a candidate variant has previously been reported to cause a disease; determine whether variants that appear in previous databases have a low frequency (*i.e.,* compatible with the observed frequency of the rare disease); determine whether loss-of-function, gain-of-function, dominant negative, haploinsufficiency, and so on are known underlying mechanisms of disease; determine whether a variant occurs in an exon and/or protein domain compatible with alteration of function; and summarize whether the candidate variants occur in similarly affected family members (pattern of inheritance and cosegregation). If a variant has been observed in the proband and other family members are tested, then the expectation is that it will exactly segregate with the disease. An example would be testing for a mutation in X-linked SCID in two brothers. The causal variant

will be present in both. When the proband is the only affected individual, then one may look to the literature; ClinVar (www.clinicalgenome.org/data-sharing/clinvar/), a database of variants with curated interpretations; and locus-specific public databases (bioinf.uta.fi/base_root/mutationdatabases.php) to determine whether the specific variant has previously been observed in another affected person. However, it is routine to find variants that have not previously been observed. Assessment of the functional consequence of a newly observed sequence variant is problematic, as there is no guarantee that it is anything more than a rare, but neutral, polymorphism. Loss-of-function mutations (*e.g.,* nonsense, frameshift, and conserved splice site mutations) have clear functional consequences. Missense substitutions are more difficult. Several methods based on sequence conservation and the chemical properties of amino acids have been developed. These are available in software, such as Sorting Intolerant From Tolerant (SIFT) (http://blocks.fhcrc.org/sift/SIFT.html), PolyPhen (http://coot.embl.de/PolyPhen/), and several others. CADD represents a class of software that creates a joint model based on integration of many of these methods.[33] All these criteria are put together in a process called *gene and variant curation.* Recommendations for scoring variants into five categories—pathogenic, likely pathogenic, variant of unknown significance, likely benign, and benign—have been given by the American College of Medical Genetics and Association for Molecular Pathology.[34]

The next step in the process is assembly of filtered and classified variants into the laboratory report. The report must be simple enough for physicians who are not experts in genomics to understand but, at the same time, must document the intermediate results required to demonstrate analytical accuracy and clinical validity. Clinical reports must contain clear nomenclature for the position and consequence of relevant variants along with appropriate indication of test and interpretive limitations. The final steps of interpretation and reporting may be facilitated by communication with the referring clinician so that there is active collaboration in arriving at a clinical diagnosis.

The final steps in bioinformatics management of NGS tests are aggregation and data sharing. Submission of deidentified cases to public-knowledge databases, such as ClinVar, will allow aggregation of variant data accompanied by sufficient clinical information to support variant classification. Once this information is accumulated in many clinical contexts, the value for patient care will be magnified beyond what could be inferred from the case data alone. Data sharing that is consistent, standardized, and collected with appropriate protections for confidentiality will be an invaluable resource for the future.

Clinical Performance of Genomics Assays

The development of specialized training programs in molecular genetics and molecular genetic pathology by the American Boards of Medical Genetics and Pathology[35] highlights the recognition by professional groups that this area of clinical testing is exceptionally complex. Although inferences made about disease diagnosis and carrier status based on direct detection of mutations are inherently categorical, data interpretation should incorporate known genotype-phenotype correlations, variable disease expression/severity, incomplete penetrance, gender-specific risk, and other available data. In the future, as DNA testing is employed in the assessment of more complex traits such as autoimmune and neoplastic diseases, genotype data will perhaps be expressed as "relative risk" and incorporate gene-gene and gene-environment interactions. The reliability of these estimates will require standard data acquisition algorithms and constant updating of population-based data.

RECOMMENDATIONS FOR USE

> **Key Concepts**
> *Principles of Molecular Diagnostics*
>
> - DNA diagnostics can play an important role in the diagnosis of specific diseases in affected individuals and in genetic risk assessment for their family members.
> - Genotyping can be used to conduct prenatal diagnoses.
> - Prenatal diagnosis may be used not only for elective termination of pregnancy but also for treatment planning.
> - Provision of genetic testing results to patients and their families carries responsibilities for sensitivity and confidentiality.

Clinically Important Applications of Next-Generation Sequencing

Molecular diagnostic techniques have a wide range of potential applications in clinical immunology. DNA diagnostic procedures are used to *(i)* perform HLA genotyping; *(ii)* analyze and monitor neoplastic

disease; *(iii)* provide identification or DNA "fingerprinting"; *(iv)* monitor bone marrow engraftment; *(v)* establish a genetic diagnosis in a symptomatic individual; *(vi)* determine the risk of occurrence of a disease in offspring; and *(vii)* to establish a prenatal diagnosis. DNA techniques are used in leukemias and lymphomas, primarily for investigation of cell lineage, proliferative clonality, and measurement of residual abnormal cells after therapy. Molecular analysis, and especially molecular cytogenetic analysis, is important in guiding initial and follow-up therapies.

Targeted Panels

When the phenotype is sufficiently circumscribed that a limited list of genes is known to account for a high percentage of cases, it may be appropriate to use a targeted gene panel as the first-round genetic diagnostic test. The reasons include assay design strategy that puts maximum emphasis on complete gene coverage; lower unit cost of testing; and reduced occurrence of secondary findings (*i.e.*, apparently pathogenic variants in genes not suspected from the primary indication for testing). But efficient use of targeted panels requires high sensitivity in the sense that most of the important disease-causing genes must have been accounted for and give a conclusive diagnosis in a large fraction of clinical cases. This situation is often not met because of the lack of specificity in clinical presentation or the very large degree of locus heterogeneity. The latter is particularly important in PIDs.

Whole-Exome/Whole-Genome Sequencing

In the past, clinical genetic testing would necessarily stop after the most likely genes had been investigated in a few targeted laboratory tests. That strategy changed in the last few years after it became possible to efficiently assess most known disease genes in a single test. Two approaches are in use today: WES and WGS.[36] WES depends on "capture" of the 1−1.5% of the genome that contains the protein-coding segments of genes. Capture is typically achieved by liquid phase hybridization followed by PCR and sequencing library construction. The rationale for WES is that most interpretable disease causing variants occur in coding sequence, and thus the sequencing is focused on the interpretable fraction of the genome. The lower unit cost of WES also allows for greater read depth with concomitantly lower error rates. Some significant limitations of WES include incomplete coverage of disease-causing genes because of inefficient capture; uneven coverage across all targeted regions such that adding more read depth inefficiently adds to poorly covered regions; poor ability to resolve structural variants; limited ability to call copy number variants; and inability to call triplet repeat mutations. WGS, especially when implemented with PCR-free library construction techniques, overcomes most of these limitations. The falling cost of WGS, especially when coupled to automated library preparation systems, holds the promise of nearly complete analysis of the genome of individuals.

Cell-Free DNA and Liquid Biopsy

It has been known for many years that there is normally a small amount of genomic DNA in the cell-free plasma fraction of blood (called *cfDNA*). It is thought that this material comes from the normal processes of cell apoptosis, particularly from leukocytes. During pregnancy, there is a significant contribution of DNA from the placenta, and thus cfDNA can be used as a biological surrogate for the fetal genome. NGS enables sampling of this DNA at very high read depth, and common chromosomal imbalances in the fetus can be detected by analysis of DNA extracted from maternal plasma. The observation of a patient who had cancer during pregnancy led to the discovery that cancer cells may also contribute to cfDNA. New genomic assays for detection of cancer recurrence, changes in mutation spectrum, and clonal expansion are rapidly arriving in clinical practice. These assays are likely to be especially useful in lymphomas and other solid tumors that have required invasive biopsies. Serial testing by these so-called liquid biopsy methods is very likely to have a large impact in immune-oncology practice.

LABORATORY STANDARDS AND REPORTING

All US laboratories providing any clinical data are subject to the regulatory requirements embodied in CLIA88.[37] CLIA88 mandates biannual laboratory inspections, quality control, quality assurance, proficiency testing, and personnel training standards. The American College of Medical Genetics has also produced guidelines for diagnostic laboratories conducting molecular genetics testing. A clear argument can be made for the clinical utility of early diagnosis for rare diseases, but demonstrating reduced cost of care or improved clinical outcome is difficult. Genomics tests, like all diagnostic testing, should be designed and developed such that the practiced test can meet the requirements of its intended use. The performance of genomic tests must be validated before they are offered for clinical diagnostic use. Critical measures of performance include sensitivity—how often the test is positive when a disease causing variant is present; specificity—how often the test is negative when a mutation is not present; "technical" positive predictive value (TPPV)—the fraction of true positives divided

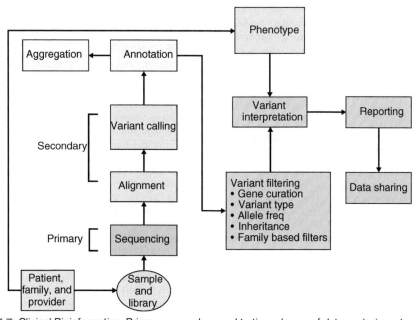

FIG. 7.7 Clinical Bioinformatics. Primary, secondary, and tertiary phases of data analysis and reporting.

by the sum of the true positive and false-positive tests; and positive and negative percent agreement with previous reference standards. These are all measures recommended by the FDA in its draft guidance for validating clinical NGS tests. New methods to test and validate bioinformatics software are also needed as the field moves forward (Fig. 7.7).

FUTURE DIRECTIONS

The next decade will bring further improvements in our ability to identify family-specific pathogenic variants for all genes that cause rare mendelian disorders, such as PIDs. Sequencing technology will continue to develop, further reducing the cost of genome analysis for individuals and families. As our understanding of the role of polymorphisms in disease risk increases, the importance of low-cost, high-throughput genotyping of standard variant panels will also increase.[38] The importance of bioinformatics in data analysis will become increasingly apparent as large amounts of individual sequence data are produced. International clinical variant databases will play an important role in both diagnosis and prognosis. New statistical approaches will be needed to exploit fully the potential of complete genome sequence for estimation of disease risk. Prospective screening of newborns for the T-cell immune deficiencies is feasible.[39,40] Although rare, these are treatable disorders whose prognosis would be altered by early diagnosis before the onset of serious infection. In aggregate, the birth incidence is sufficient to merit screening if the techniques could be interfaced with current state screening programs. Screening for premalignant genotypic changes in peripheral blood might also be a reality one day. Careful clinical studies, including examination of the costs and benefits of mass screening programs, will be essential.

On the Horizon

- Routine diagnosis of >300 primary immunodeficiencies by whole-genome sequencing
- Rapid discovery of new primary immune deficiency genes by whole-genome sequencing in individual families
- Preconceptional screening to identify carrier status for thousands of genetic disorders
- Noninvasive prenatal screening of fetal DNA in maternal blood for copy number abnormalities and mutations

---

TRANSLATIONAL RESEARCH AND CLINICAL APPLICATION

DNA sequencing technology is evolving very rapidly, and we can anticipate additional technical platforms to become available over the next decade. Massive increases in sequence output, speed of sequencing, increases in read length, and more efficient bioinformatics methods will fuel further reductions in cost. Complete genome sequencing will likely become a first-line medical test for the diagnosis of most suspected genetic disorders, including the PIDs. Gene identification in single families with previously undescribed immune deficiencies will become routine. Personal complete genome sequencing for preconceptual genetic screening in the general population will become available and will impact risk counseling for thousands of patients with autosomal recessive and X-linked disorders. By analysis of either free DNA in maternal serum or circulating fetal cells, complete genome sequencing will provide a comprehensive testing platform for noninvasive prenatal diagnosis. Incorporation of other methods, such as RNA sequencing, will undoubtedly become part of routine functional assessment of suspected pathogenic variants. Single-cell sequencing technology promises to give much greater detail on the beautifully complicated problem of immune cell heterogeneity. Although single-cell sequencing has not yet been shown to have role in clinical diagnostics, it may present the next step in the long-term goal of understanding immunological diseases at the cellular level.

REFERENCES

1. Raje N, Dinakar C. Overview of immunodeficiency disorders. *Immunol Allergy Clin North Am.* 2015;35:599−623.
2. Picard C, Al-Herz W, Bousfiha A, et al. Primary immunodeficiency diseases: an update on the classification from the international union of immunological societies expert committee for primary immunodeficiency. *J Clin Immunol.* 2015;2015(35):696−726.
3. Genomes Project C, Auton A, Brooks LD, et al. A global reference for human genetic variation. *Nature.* 2015;526:68−74.
4. International HapMap C, Altshuler DM, Gibbs RA, et al. Integrating common and rare genetic variation in diverse human populations. *Nature.* 2010;467:52−58.
5. Picard C, Fischer A. Contribution of high-throughput DNA sequencing to the study of primary immunodeficiencies. *Eur J Immunol.* 2014;44:2854−2861.
6. Platt C, Geha RS, Chou J. Gene hunting in the genomic era: approaches to diagnostic dilemmas in patients with

primary immunodeficiencies. *J Allergy Clin Immunol.* 2014; 134:262−268.

7. MacArthur DG, Manolio TA, Dimmock DP, et al. Guidelines for investigating causality of sequence variants in human disease. *Nature.* 2014;508:469−476.

8. de Jong H. Visualizing DNA domains and sequences by microscopy: a fifty-year history of molecular cytogenetics. *Genome.* 2003;46:943−946.

9. Coughlin 2nd CR, Scharer GH, Shaikh TH. Clinical impact of copy number variation analysis using high-resolution microarray technologies: advantages, limitations and concerns. *Genome Med.* 2012;4:80.

10. Martin CL, Kirkpatrick BE, Ledbetter DH. Copy number variants, aneuploidies, and human disease. *Clin Perinatol.* 2015;42:227−242, vii.

11. Shendure J, Akey JM. The origins, determinants, and consequences of human mutations. *Science.* 2015;349: 1478−1483.

12. Mullaney JM, Mills RE, Pittard WS, et al. Small insertions and deletions (INDELs) in human genomes. *Hum Mol Genet.* 2010;19:R131−R136.

13. Budworth H, McMurray CT. A brief history of triplet repeat diseases. *Methods Mol Biol.* 2013;1010:3−17.

14. Fragouli E, Wells D, Delhanty JD. Chromosome abnormalities in the human oocyte. *Cytogenet Genome Res.* 2011;133:107−118.

15. Jones KT, Lane SI. Molecular causes of aneuploidy in mammalian eggs. *Development.* 2013;140:3719−3730.

16. Campbell CD, Eichler EE. Properties and rates of germline mutations in humans. *Trends Genet.* 2013;29:575−584.

17. Segurel L, Wyman MJ, Przeworski M. Determinants of mutation rate variation in the human germline. *Annu Rev Genomics Hum Genet.* 2014;15:47−70.

18. Belmont JW. Genetic control of X inactivation and processes leading to X-inactivation skewing. *Am J Hum Genet.* 1996;58:1101−1108.

19. Liehr T, Weise A, Hamid AB, et al. Multicolor FISH methods in current clinical diagnostics. *Expert Rev Mol Diagn.* 2013;13:251−255.

20. Barrett MT, Scheffer A, Ben-Dor A, et al. Comparative genomic hybridization using oligonucleotide microarrays and total genomic DNA. *Proc Natl Acad Sci USA.* 2004; 101:17765−17770.

21. Lipshutz RJ, Fodor SP, Gingeras TR, et al. High density synthetic oligonucleotide arrays. *Nat Genet.* 1999;21:20−24.

22. Peiffer DA, Le JM, Steemers FJ, et al. High-resolution genomic profiling of chromosomal aberrations using Infinium whole-genome genotyping. *Genome Res.* 2006; 16(9):1136−1148.

23. Cooper GM, Zerr T, Kidd JM, et al. Systematic assessment of copy number variant detection via genome-wide SNP genotyping. *Nat Genet.* 2008;40:1199−1203.

24. Fan JB, Chee MS, Gunderson KL. Highly parallel genomic assays. *Nat Rev Genet.* 2006;7:632−644.

25. Kennedy GC, Matsuzaki H, Dong S, et al. Large-scale genotyping of complex DNA. *Nat Biotechnol.* 2003;21: 1233−1237.

26. Gunderson KL, Steemers FJ, Lee G, et al. A genome-wide scalable SNP genotyping assay using microarray technology. *Nat Genet.* 2005;37:549−554.

27. Strom CM. Mutation detection, interpretation, and applications in the clinical laboratory setting. *Mutat Res.* 2005; 573:160−167.

28. Bentley DR, Balasubramanian S, Swerdlow HP, et al. Accurate whole human genome sequencing using reversible terminator chemistry. *Nature.* 2008;456:53−59.

29. Rothberg JM, Hinz W, Rearick TM, et al. An integrated semiconductor device enabling non-optical genome sequencing. *Nature.* 2011;475:348−352.

30. Goodwin S, McPherson JD, McCombie WR. Coming of age: ten years of next-generation sequencing technologies. *Nat Rev Genet.* 2016;17:333−351.

31. Stoloff DH, Wanunu M. Recent trends in nanopores for biotechnology. *Curr Opin Biotechnol.* 2013;24: 699−704.

32. Roller E, Ivakhno S, Lee S, et al. Canvas: versatile and scalable detection of copy number variants. *Bioinformatics.* 2016;32:2375−2377.

33. Kircher M, Witten DM, Jain P, et al. A general framework for estimating the relative pathogenicity of human genetic variants. *Nat Genet.* 2014;46:310−315.

34. Richards S, Aziz N, Bale S, et al. Standards and guidelines for the interpretation of sequence variants: a joint consensus recommendation of the american college of medical genetics and genomics and the association for molecular pathology. *Genet Med.* 2015; 17:405−424.

35. Byers PH. Molecular genetic pathology. Coming of age in the molecular world. *Am J Pathol.* 1999;155:673−674.

36. Prokop JW, May T, Strong K, et al. Genome sequencing in the clinic: The past, present and future of genomic medicine. *Physiol Genomics*; 2018. https://doi.org/10.1152/physiolgenomics. 00046.2018.

37. Rivers PA, Dobalian A, Germinario FA. A review and analysis of the clinical laboratory improvement amendment of 1988: compliance plans and enforcement policy. *Health Care Manage Rev.* 2005;30:93−102.

38. Worthey EA, Mayer AN, Syverson GD, et al. Making a definitive diagnosis: successful clinical application of whole exome sequencing in a child with intractable inflammatory bowel disease. *Genet Med.* 2011;13: 255−262.

39. Routes JM, Grossman WJ, Verbsky J, et al. Statewide newborn screening for severe T-cell lymphopenia. *JAMA.* 2009;302:2465−2470.

40. King JR, Hammerström L. Newborn screening for primary immunodeficiency diseases: History, current and future practice. *J Clin Immunol.* 2018;38:56−66.

Characteristics of Selected CD Molecules

THOMAS A. FLEISHER

CD Molecule	Predominant Distribution	Identity/Function
CD1a—e	Thymocytes, subset of lymphocytes, antigen-presenting cells	MHC class I—like molecules; presentation of nonpeptide antigens to T cells; thymic T-cell development
CD2	T cells	Binds to LFA-3; receptor for CD48; T-cell activation; adhesion
CD3	T cells	T-cell signaling complex; associated with TCR
CD4	T-cell subset	TCR coreceptor; interacts with MHC class II molecules on antigen-presenting cells; identifies T cells with helper function; signal transduction
CD5	Most T cells, thymocytes, B-cell subset	Binds to CD72; regulation of cell proliferation/activation; identifies B-1 B-cell subset
CD6	Thymocytes, T cells, B-cell subset	Binds CD166 (ALCAM); adhesion; mediates binding of developing thymocytes with thymic epithelial cells; thymic development; T-cell activation
CD7	Pluripotent hematopoietic cells, thymocytes, T cells	T-cell and NK-cell development
CD8	T-cell subset	TCR coreceptor; interacts with MHC class I molecules on antigen-presenting cells; identifies T cells with cytotoxic function
CD10	B cells	Neutral endopeptidase; enkephalinase; B-cell development; common acute lymphoblastic leukemia antigen (CALLA), neutrophils
CD11a	Leukocytes	α-chain of LFA-1; pairs with CD18; interacts with ICAM; adhesion and cellular migration
CD11b	Monocytes, granulocytes, NK cells	α-chain of complement receptor type 3 (CR3); pairs with CD18; adhesion molecule
CD11c	Monocytes, granulocytes, NK cells	α-chain of complement receptor type 4 (CR4); pairs with CD18; adhesion molecule
CD13	Hematopoietic stem cells, immature and mature myeloid and monocyte elements	Appears before CD33 during myeloid differentiation
CD14	Granulocytes, monocytes/macrophages	Receptor for LPS/LPB complex; myeloid differentiation antigen; cell activation
CD15	Neutrophils, eosinophils, monocytes, basophil subset	Sialyl Lewis X antigen, plays a role in cell adhesion, defective in leukocyte adhesion deficiency type 2

Continued

CD Molecule	Predominant Distribution	Identity/Function
CD16a,b	NK cells, monocytes/macrophages, neutrophils	FcγRIIIA and FcγRIIIB (low-affinity IgG receptor type III); phagocytosis; ADCC
CD18	Leukocytes	β-chain of $β_2$-integrin molecules, including LFA-1, CR3, and CR4; pairs with CD11a, b, and c
CD19	B cells	BCR coreceptor; signal transduction; complexes with CD21, expressed pre-B cells
CD20	B cells	Role in B-cell activation/differentiation
CD21	B cells; follicular dendritic cells	Complement receptor type 2 (CR2): C3d receptor; B-cell coreceptor subunit; EBV receptor
CD22	B cells	Associates with BCR; signaling; regulation of B-cell activation; adhesion
CD23	B cells, macrophages, eosinophils, platelets, follicular dendritic cells	FcεRII; (low-affinity IgE receptor), activated B cells
CD24	Leukocytes	Heat-stable antigen; costimulation; adhesion
CD25	Activated T cells and B cells	α-chain of IL-2 receptor, low-affinity IL-2 binding; signaling for cell proliferation/differentiation
CD26	Activated T cells and B cells; macrophages	Dipeptidyl peptidase; role in extracellular adhesion; cell activation
CD27	T cells; B-cell subset	Costimulation; T-cell proliferation; memory B cells
CD28	T cells	Binds B7-1 (CD80) and B7-2 (CD86); T-cell costimulation; signal transduction
CD29	Leukocytes	Integrin $β_1$-chain; pairs with CD49a–CD49f to form VLA-1–VLA-6 integrins, respectively; adhesion; signal transduction; development
CD30	Activated B cells and T cells	Binds to CD153; T-cell activation/regulation/differentiation, Reed-Sternberg cells
CD31	Monocytes, granulocytes, platelets, endothelial cells, B cells Recent thymic emigrants	PECAM-1; binds to CD38; adhesion; signal transduction
CD32	B cells, monocytes/macrophages, granulocytes, eosinophils	FcgRII (low-affinity IgG receptor type II) phagocytosis; ADCC; B-cell regulation
CD33	Myeloid progenitors, granulocytes	Binds sialic acid
CD34	Hematopoietic progenitor cells; capillary endothelium	Mucosialin; binds to CD62L; adhesion
CD35	Leukocytes; erythrocytes	Complement receptor 1 (CR1); C3b and C4b receptor; phagocytosis
CD36	Monocytes/macrophages; endothelium; platelets	Binds oxidized LDL; scavenger receptor; binds apoptotic cells; adhesion and endocytic receptor; GPIIIb; platelet adhesion and aggregation
CD38	NK cells; T-cell and B-cell subsets; monocytes	Binds CD31; cyclase; hydrolase; cell activation
CD40	B cells; antigen-presenting cells	Binds CD154 (CD40 ligand); B-cell proliferation, differentiation, and survival; T-cell costimulation
CD41	Megakaryocytes/platelets	Glycoprotein IIb; a IIb integrin chain; binds fibronectin, fibrinogen, von Willebrand factor, thrombospondin; extracellular adhesion; platelet aggregation

CD Molecule	Predominant Distribution	Identity/Function
CD43	Leukocytes (except resting B cells)	Leukocyte sialoglycoprotein; may bind CD54; signal transduction; adhesion; antiadhesion
CD44	Leukocytes; memory T cells; erythrocytes	Binds hyaluronan (H-CAM), collagen, fibronectin, laminin, osteopontin; extra- and intercellular adhesion; T-cell costimulation; leukocyte homing
CD45	Leukocytes (pan-leukocyte marker)	Protein tyrosine phosphatase; cell differentiation; lymphocyte signal transduction and activation
CD45RA	Naive T-cell marker (in conjunction with CD62L); B cells, monocytes	CD45 isoform
CD45RB	B-cell and T-cell subsets, monocytes/macrophages, granulocytes	CD45 isoform
CD45RO	Memory and activated T cells; B cells, monocytes/macrophages	CD45 isoform
CD46	Hematopoietic cells	Membrane cofactor protein (MCP); binds to C3b and C4b and regulates complement pathway
CD47R	Leukocytes; endothelium	Integrin-associated protein (IAP); leukocyte migration, extravasation, and activation
CD48	Leukocytes (not neutrophils)	Binds CD2; adhesion; costimulation
CD49a–f	Various distributions	Integrin a1–a6 chain; binds to CD29 to form VLA-1 to VLA-6; binds extracellular matrix components such as fibronectin, laminin, collagen (CD49D binds VCAM-1, fibronectin, MAdCAM-1, invasin); lymphocyte homing; extracellular adhesion; embryonic development
CD50	Thymocytes, B cells, T cells, monocytes, granulocytes	ICAM-3; adhesion
CD51	Platelets/megakaryocytes, granulocytes, monocytes, T cells	Integrin α-chain; associates with CD61; binds vitronectin, fibronectin, fibrinogen; extracellular adhesion; T-cell costimulation; epithelial inflammatory response
CD52	Leukocytes	GPI linked, signaling, defined by CAMPATH-1
CD54	Broad distribution; increased on activated leukocytes	ICAM-1; binds LFA-1; adhesion; leukocyte transendothelial migration, rhinovirus receptor
CD55	Hematopoietic cells and some nonhematopoietic cells	Decay accelerating factor (DAF); binds complement fragment C3b; regulation of complement activation
CD56	NK cells, NK-T cells	NKH-1; adhesion
CD57	NK cells, T-cell subset, B cells, monocytes	Oligosaccharide expressed on cell surface glycoproteins
CD58	Hematopoietic cells and non-hematopoietic cells	LFA-3; binds CD2; adhesion; lymphocyte coactivation
CD59	Hematopoietic cells and non-hematopoietic cells	Binds complement components C8 and C9 and regulates assembly of complement membrane attack complex
CD61	Platelets/megakaryocytes, macrophages	Integrin β_3 subunit; associates with CD41 or CD51

Continued

CD Molecule	Predominant Distribution	Identity/Function
CD62E	Endothelium	ELAM-1 or E-selection; binds sialyl-Lewis X; adhesion; mediates rolling interaction of neutrophils on endothelium and neutrophil extravasation
CD62L	B cells, T cells, monocytes, NK cells	LECAM-1, LAM-1 (or L-selectin); binds CD34 and GlyCAM; adhesion; mediates rolling interactions with endothelium and call extravasation
CD62P	Platelets/megakaryocytes, endothelium	P-selectin; binds sialyl-Lewis X; mediates interaction of platelets with neutrophils and monocytes; mediates rolling interaction of neutrophils with endothelium
CD64	Monocytes/macrophages, mature neutrophils	$Fc\gamma R1$ (high-affinity IgG receptor)
CD65	Neutrophils, eosinophils, basophils monocyte subset, CD56 bright NK cells	During myeloid differentiation it appears after myeloperoxidase, appears to be the ligand for CD62L
CD66c	Differentiating myeloid cells peaks at promyelocyte stage, subpopulation of monocytes	Member of the carcinoembryonic antigen (CEA) family
CD68	Monocytes/macrophages	Macrosialin; early activation antigen; role in phagocytic activity
CD69	Activated T cells, B cells, macrophages, NK cells	Early activation antigen; costimulation
CD70	Activated B cells and T cells; macrophages	Binds to CD27; costimulation
CD71	Activated leukocytes, erythroid precursors	Transferrin receptor; cell activation
CD72	B cells	Ligand for CD5; B-cell activation and differentiation; costimulation
CD73	B-cell and T-cell subsets	Ecto-5′ nucleotidase; allows nucleoside uptake
CD74	MHC class II−expressing cells	MHC class II−associated invariant chain; involved in antigen processing and peptide presentation in antigen-presenting cells
CD77	Germinal center B cells	Entering apoptosis
CD79a,b	B cells	Iga, Igb; components of BCR complex that mediate signal transduction
CD80	Monocytes/macrophages, dendritic cells, activated B cells	B7-1; ligand for CD28 and CTLA-4; T-cell interaction with antigen-presenting cells; costimulation
CD81	Lymphocytes	Associates with CD19 and CD21 to form B-cell coreceptor complex; costimulation; adhesion
CD86	Monocytes, activated B cells	B7-2; ligand for CD28 and CTLA-4; T-cell interaction with antigen-presenting cells; costimulation
CD87	Granulocytes; monocytes/macrophages, activated T cells	Urokinase plasminogen activator receptor
CD88	Granulocytes, macrophages, mast cells	Complement component fragment C5a receptor
CD89	Monocytes/macrophages, granulocytes, B-cell and T-cell subsets	$Fc\alpha R$ (IgA receptor)

CD Molecule	Predominant Distribution	Identity/Function
CD91	Monocytes	α_2-macroglobulin receptor
CD94	NK cells, T-cell subset	Inhibits killing
CD95	Broad distribution	Fas or APO-1; induces apoptosis after being bound by Fas ligand
CD97	Activated B and T cells, monocytes, PMN	Activation antigen
CD102	Resting lymphocytes, monocytes, endothelial cells	ICAM-2; binds LFA-1 (CD11a/CD18); adhesion; T-cell costimulation
CD103	Intraepithelial lymphocytes, T-cell subset	αE integrin; T-cell development and costimulation
CD104	Epithelial cells, Schwann cells	β_4-integrin; epidermal adhesion to basement membrane
CD105	Endothelial cells, bone marrow cell subset, activated macrophages	Endoglin; adhesion
CD106	Endothelial cells	VCAM-1; ligand for VLA-4; lymphocyte adhesion; embryonic development
CD107a,b	Epithelial cells, subsets of monocytes, granulocytes, and lymphocytes	LAMP-1 and LAMP-2; adhesion
CD110	Hematopoietic stem cells, megakaryocytes, platelets	Thrombopoietin receptor; megakaryocyte proliferation and differentiation
CD114	Granulocytes	G-CSF receptor; regulates granulopoiesis
CD115	Monocytes/macrophages	M-CSF receptor; cell differentiation
CD116	Monocytes, neutrophils, eosinophils	GM-CSF a chain receptor; cell differentiation
CD117	Hematopoietic progenitors, mast cells	c-*kit*; stem cell factor (SCF) receptor; hematopoietic cell differentiation
CD118	Broad distribution	Type 1 interferon (interferon-α/β) receptor
CD119	Broad distribution	Interferon-γ receptor
CD120a	Hematopoietic cells, nonhematopoietic cells, myeloid cells	TNF receptor type I; signal transduction; apoptosis
CD120b	Hematopoietic cells, nonhematopoietic cells, myeloid cells	TNF receptor type II; signal transduction; apoptosis
CD121a	Thymocytes, T-cell subset, fibroblasts, epithelial cells, and brain cells	IL-1 receptor type I; signal transduction
CD121b	T-cell subset, myeloid cell subsets	IL-1 receptor type II
CD122	NK cells, T-cell and B-cell subset	IL-2 and IL-15 receptor β chain; signal transduction; regulation of lymphocyte development, differentiation, activation, and proliferation
CD123	Bone marrow stem cells, granulocytes, monocytes, megakaryocytes	IL-3 receptor α chain; cell development and differentiation

Continued

CD Molecule	Predominant Distribution	Identity/Function
CD124	Mature B cells and T cells, hematopoietic precursor cells	IL-4 receptor; signal transduction; lymphocyte development, activation, differentiation, and proliferation
CD125	Eosinophils, basophils, B-cell subset	IL-5 receptor; eosinophil and B-cell growth and differentiation
CD126	Activated B cells, plasma cells, T cells, granulocytes, monocytes/macrophages; also expressed on epithelial cells, fibroblasts, hepatocytes, and neural cells	IL-6 receptor α chain; regulation of B-cell and T-cell differentiation and function; hematopoiesis
CD127	Bone marrow lymphoid precursors, pro-B cells, T-cell precursors, T-cell subset, monocytes	IL-7 receptor α chain; signal transduction; B-cell and T-cell proliferation and differentiation
CD128	Neutrophils, basophils, T-cell subset	IL-8 receptor; neutrophil activation and migration
CD129	T cells	IL-9 receptor α chain; T-cell proliferation
CD130	Broad distribution	IL-6 receptor β chain (with CD126); signal transduction
CD131	Lymphocytes, granulocytes, monocytes	IL-3, IL-5, and GM-CSF receptor; common β chain; signal transduction; see CD123 and CD125
CD132	Lymphocytes	Common γ chain of high-affinity receptor for IL-2 (with CD25 and CD122), IL-4 (with CD124), IL-7 (with CD127), IL-9 (with CD129), and IL-15 (with CD122) receptors; signal transduction
CD134	Activated T cells	OX-40 antigen of TNFR superfamily (binds OX-40 ligand); T cell-B cell interaction and T-cell costimulation
CD135	Lymphoid and myeloid cell progenitor subsets	Flt3 ligand receptor; development of myeloid and lymphoid progenitors
CD137	Activated T cells	4-1BB; binds 4-1BB ligand and extracellular matrix components; T cell-B cell interaction and T-cell costimulation; extracellular adhesion; signal transduction
CD138	B-cell subset, plasma cells, epithelial cells	Syndecan-1; binds interstitial matrix proteins; B cell-matrix interactions
CD140a,b	Endothelial cells	PDGF receptor α and β chain; embryonic development; signal transduction; chemotaxis
CD141	Endothelium	Thrombomodulin (binds thrombin); regulates coagulation
CD142	Endothelium	Tissue factor; binds plasma factors VII/VIIa; hemostasis, coagulation, and angiogenesis
CD143	Endothelium	Angiotensin-converting enzyme (ACE); binds angiotensin 1; regulates blood pressure
CD144	Endothelium	VE-cadherin; cell-cell adhesion; maintenance of endothelium integrity
CD146	Activated T-cell subset	Mel-CAM, adhesion molecule during development

CD Molecule	Predominant Distribution	Identity/Function
CD150	T-cell and B-cell subsets	Surface lymphocyte activation marker (SLAM); B cell-T cell interaction; costimulation
CD151	Not defined	PETA-3; regulates platelet aggregation and mediator release
CD152	Activated T cells	CTLA-4; binds B7-1 (CD80) and B7-2 (CD86); T-cell costimulation—negative signal
CD153	T cells	CD30 ligand; T-cell activation, differentiation, and regulation
CD154	Activated T cells	CD40 ligand; T-cell costimulation
CD156a	Leukocytes, B cells	Transmembrane glycoprotein; disintegrin and metalloproteinase domain (ADAM) family member; leukocyte adhesion and protease function; infiltration of myelomonocytic cells
CD156b	Broad distribution	TNF-α-converting enzyme (TACE); disintegrin and metalloproteinase domain (ADAM) family member; cleaves TNF and transforming growth factor-α from cell surface, thereby releasing soluble form
CD158	NK cells	Killer immunoglobulin-like receptors (KIR); family of molecules that inhibit NK cytotoxic activity
CD159a	NK cells	NKG2A (natural killer cell lectin-like receptor)
CD161	NK cells	Natural killer cell receptor-P1; target cell recognition; NK-cell activation
CD162	Granulocyte and T-cell subsets	P-selectin glycoprotein ligand-1 (PSGL-1); adhesion
CD166	Activated T cells, B cells	ALCAM; binds CD6; T-cell activation; thymocyte development
CD167a	Epithelial cells	Discoidin domain receptor 1 (DDR1); tyrosine kinase receptor; binds to collagen; cell-cell contact and adhesion
CD178	Activated T cells; various tissue cells	FAS ligand (ligand for CD95); binding to FAS triggers apoptosis
CD179a	Pro-B and pre-B cells	VpreB; forms surrogate light chain with CD179b; early B-cell differentiation
CD179b	Pro-B and pre-B cells	λ5; forms surrogate light chain with CD179a; early B-cell differentiation
CD180	B cells	RP105; toll-like receptor family; regulates B-cell recognition and signaling of LPS
CD183	Effector/memory T cells, NK cells, eosinophils	CXCR3 receptor for interferon-inducible chemokines IP10, Mig, and I-TAC; chemotactic migration of effector T cells into areas of inflammation
CD184	Leukocytes; hematopoietic progenitors	CXCR4 receptor for chemokines such as stromal cell–derived factor 1 (SDF-1) (fusin); chemotaxis; HIV-1 coreceptor
CD195	Broad distribution; myeloid cells, lymphocytes, T lymphocytes, neurons, epithelium, endothelium	CCR5 receptor for chemokines such as macrophage inflammatory proteins, MIP-1a and MIP-1b, and RANTES; chemotaxis; HIV-1 coreceptor
CDw197	Lymphoid tissues, B cells, T-cell subset	CCR7 chemokine receptor; chemotaxis; T-cell homing and migration
CD201	Endothelial cells	Protein C receptor; coagulation

Continued

CD Molecule	Predominant Distribution	Identity/Function
CD203c	Mast cells, basophils	Member of the ectonucleotide pyrophosphatase/phosphodiesterase enzymes
CD204	Myeloid cells, monocytes/macrophages	Macrophage scavenger receptor-1 (MSR1); mediates binding, internalization, and processing of various negatively charged macromolecules
CD206	Dendritic cells, macrophages, myeloid cells, endothelial cells	Mannose receptor, C type 1; binds microorganisms; phagocytosis
CD207	Dendritic cells, Langerhans cells	Langerin; mannose receptor; phagocytosis and internalization of antigen for processing
CD208	Dendritic cells	DC-LAMP
CD209	Dendritic cells	DC-SIGN
CDw210	Broad distribution	IL–10 receptor α and β chain
CD212	T cells, NK cells	IL-12 receptor β_1 chain
CD213a1,a2	Lymphocytes, bronchial epithelial and smooth muscle cells	IL-13 receptor α_1 and α_2 chains
CDw217	Activated T-cell subset	IL-17; cytotoxic T-lymphocyte–associated serine esterase 8; stimulates cell activation; induces osteoclast differentiation factor (ODF)
CD220	Broad distribution	Insulin receptor; stimulates glucose uptake
CD molecule	Predominant distribution	Identity/function
CD221	Broad distribution	Insulin-like growth factor 1 receptor; cell signaling, activation, and differentiation
CD222	Broad distribution	Mannose-6-phosphate receptor; insulin-like growth factor 2 receptor
CD226	NK cells, platelets, monocytes, T-cell subset	Platelet and T-cell activation antigen 1 (PTA1); adhesion
CD233–241	Erythrocytes	Various erythrocyte membrane antigens, including blood group–associated glycoproteins
CD242	Erythrocytes	ICAM-4
CD246	T cells	TCR or CD3 ζ chain; associated with TCR and CD3; couples TCR recognition with T-cell signaling
CD247	T cells	T cells ζ chain of the TcR
CD252	Activated B cells	OX40 ligand
CD253	Activated T cells	TRAIL, death receptor
CD254	Activated T cells, LN and BM stroma	RANK ligand
CD256	Monocytes, macrophages	APRIL, binds TACI and BCMA
CD257	Activated monocytes	BLyS, BAFF, binds TACI, BCMA, BAFFR, induces B-cell proliferation
CD261	Activated T cells, peripheral leukocytes	TRAIL-R2, DR5, death receptor
CD262	Peripheral lymphocytes	TRAIL-R1, DR4, death receptor
CD263	Peripheral lymphocytes	TRAIL-R3, DcR1, death receptor

CD Molecule	Predominant Distribution	Identity/Function
CD264	Peripheral lymphocytes	TRAIL-R4, DcR2, death receptor
CD265	Broad distribution	RANK
CD267	B cells, activated T cells	TACI
CD268	B cells	BAFFR, binds BLys, mature B-cell survival
CD269	Mature B cells	BCMA, binds APRIL and BAFF, B-cell survival and proliferation
CD275	B cells, dendritic cells, monocytes	ICOSL, costimulation, cytokine production
CD278	Activated T cells	ICOS, T-cell costimulation

ADCC, antibody-dependent cellular cytotoxicity; *ALCAM,* activated leukocyte cell adhesion molecule; *APRIL,* a proliferation-inducing ligand; *BCMA,* B-cell maturation antigen; *BCR,* B-cell receptor for antigen; *DC,* dendritic cell; *CTLA,* cytotoxic T-lymphocyte antigen; *EBV,* Epstein-Barr virus; *ELAM,* endothelial leukocyte adhesion molecule; *G-CSF,* granulocyte-colony stimulating factor; *GM-CSF,* granulocyte macrophage-colony stimulating factor; *GPI,* glycosyl-phosphatidylinositol; *HIV,* human immunodeficiency virus; *ICAM,* intercellular adhesion molecule; *ICOS,* inducible T-cell costimulator; *Ig,* immunoglobulin; IL, interleukin; *LAM,* leukocyte adhesion molecule; *LAMP,* latent membrane protein; *LDL,* low-density lipoproteins; *LECAM,* lymphocyte endothelial cell adhesion molecule; *LFA,* lymphocyte function antigen; *LPB,* lipopolysaccharide-binding protein; *LPS,* lipopolysaccharide; *MAdCAM-1,* mucosal addressin cell adhesion molecule-1; *M-CSF,* macrophage-colony stimulating factor; *MHC,* major histocompatibility complex; *NK cells,* natural killer cells; *PDGF,* platelet-derived growth factor; *PECAM,* platelet endothelial cell adhesion molecule; *PETA,* platelet-endothelial cell tetraspan antigen; *PMN,* polymorphonuclear neutrophil; *SIGN,* specific intercellular adhesion molecule—grabbing nonintegrin; *TACI,* transmembrane activator and CAML interactor; *TCR,* T-cell receptor for antigen; *TNF,* tumor necrosis factor; *TNFR,* tumor necrosis factor receptor; *TRAIL,* TNF-related apoptosis—inducing ligand; *VCAM,* vascular cellular adhesion molecule; *VLA,* very late antigen.

This list was adapted from the results of the Eighth International Workshop on Human Leukocyte Differentiation Antigens (HLDA8) held in Adelaide, Australia, in December 2004 (Proceedings of the Eighth International Workshop on Human Leukocyte Differentiation Antigens. December 12—16, 2004. Adelaide, Australia. Cell Immunol 2005;236[1—2]:1—187). Engel P, Boumsell L, Balderas R, et al. CD nomenclature 2015: human leukocyte differentiation antigen workshops as a driving force in immunology. J Immunol 2015;195:4555—4563.

Laboratory Reference Values in Human Immunology

THOMAS A. FLEISHER

Age of Healthy Donors	IgG g/L	IgG$_1$ g/L	IgG$_2$ g/L	IgG$_3$ g/L	IgG$_4$ g/L	IgA g/L	IgA$_1$ g/L	IgA$_2$ g/L	IgM g/L
0–<5 months	1.00–3.34	0.56–2.15	≤0.82	0.076–0.823	≤0.198	0.07–0.37	0.10–0.34	0.004–0.055	0.26–1.22
5–<9 months	1.64–5.88	1.02–3.69	≤0.89	0.119–0.740	≤0.208	0.16–0.50	0.14–0.41	0.015–0.062	0.32–1.32
9–<15 months	2.46–9.04	1.60–5.62	0.24–0.98	0.173–0.637	≤0.220	0.27–0.66	0.20–0.50	0.028–0.070	0.40–1.43
15–<24 months	3.13–11.70	2.09–7.24	0.35–1.05	0.219–0.550	≤0.230	0.36–0.79	0.24–0.58	0.039–0.077	0.46–1.52
2–<4 years	2.95–11.56	1.58–7.21	0.39–1.76	0.170–0.847	0.004–0.491	0.27–2.46	0.16–1.62	0.013–0.311	0.37–1.84
4–<7 years	3.86–14.70	2.09–9.02	0.44–3.16	0.108–0.949	0.008–0.819	0.29–2.56	0.17–1.87	0.011–0.391	0.37–2.24
7–<10 years	4.62–16.82	2.53–10.19	0.54–4.35	0.085–1.02	0.010–1.087	0.34–2.74	0.21–2.21	0.014–0.480	0.38–2.51
10–<13 years	5.03–17.19	2.80–10.30	0.66–5.02	0.115–1.05	0.010–1.219	0.42–2.95	0.27–2.50	0.026–0.534	0.41–2.55
13–<16 years	5.09–15.80	2.89–9.34	0.82–5.16	0.200–1.03	0.007–1.217	0.52–3.19	0.36–2.75	0.047–0.551	0.45–2.44
16–<18 years	4.87–13.27	2.83–7.72	0.98–4.86	0.313–0.976	0.003–1.110	0.60–3.37	0.44–2.89	0.066–0.543	0.49–2.01
≥18 years	7.67–15.90	3.41–8.94	1.71–6.32	0.184–1.06	0.024–1.210	0.61–3.56	0.50–3.14	0.097–1.560	0.37–2.86

Immunoglobulin (Ig) levels were assessed in serum by nephelometry, and data were statistically analyzed for the mid-95% confidence interval. For total IgG and IgG subclass quantitation, data from 156 pediatric and 92 adult donors were used; for total IgA quantitation, data from 201 pediatric and 99 adult donors were used; for IgA subclasses, data from 119 pediatric and 99 adult donors were used; and for IgM quantitation, data from 212 pediatric and 401 adult donors were used at Mayo Medical Laboratories.

Age	Gender	Geometric Mean	Upper 95% Confidence Limit
6–14 years	M	42.7	527
	F	43.3	344
15–24 years	M	33.6	447
	F	18.6	262
25–34 years	M	16.8	275
	F	16.6	216
35–44 years	M	21.7	242
	F	19.3	206
45–54 years	M	19.2	254
	F	13.3	177
55–64 years	M	21.3	354
	F	11.7	148
65–74 years	M	21.2	248
	F	11.5	122
>75 years	M	18.4	219
	F	9.2	124
6–75 years	all M	22.9	317
	all F	14.7	189

Data were generated using individuals with negative skin prick tests (i.e., house dust mite, Bermuda grass, tree mix, weed mix, mold mix). From Barbee RA, Halonen M, Lebowitz M, Burrows B. Distribution of IgE in a community population sample: correlations with age, sex, and allergen skin test reactivity. J Allergy Clin Immunol 1981;68(2): 106–11, with permission.

Surface Antigens	Percent Positive	Cells/mm^3
T Cells		
CD3	60–83.5%	714–2266
CD5	60–83.5%	723–2276
CD2	77.5–94%	817–2496
CD7	74–96.0%	775–2536
CD3/CD4	32–62%	359–1565
CD3/CD8	11–35%	178–853
CD4/CD45RO	10–44%	173–916
CD4/CD45RA	4–21%	55–593
CD8/CD45RO	1.5–11.5%	36–273
CD8/CD45RA	2.5–20.5%	44–405
CD3/CD8/CD28	9.5–26%	126–600
CD8/CD57	≤30.0%	≤521
CD3/HLA-DR	≤19.5%	≤450
CD3/CD25	11–40%	155–905
B Cells		
CD20	3–19%	59–329
CD19	3–19%	61–321
CD20/CD5	0.5–9.5%	14–159
CD20/CD23	1–14%	27–229
CD20/CD27	1–3.5%	12–68
NK Cells		
CD3$^-$/CD16$^+$/CD56$^+$	6–35%	126–729
Lymphocytes	17–41%	1173–2640

Data generated in the Flow Cytometry Section, Immunology Service, DLM, CC, NIH, Bethesda, MD. The 95% confidence interval for the WBC is 4300–9200/mm^3.

T Cells						
CD3			**CD4**		**CD8**	
Age	**Percent positive**	**Cells/mm³**	**Percent positive**	**Cells/mm³**	**Percent positive**	**Cells/mm³**
0–3 mo	53–84	2500–5500	35–64	1600–4000	12–28	560–1700
3–6 mo	51–77	2500–5600	35–56	1800–4000	12–23	590–1600
6–12 mo	49–76	1900–5900	31–56	1400–4300	12–24	500–1700
1–2 yr	53–75	2100–6200	32–51	1300–4300	14–30	620–2000
2–6 yr	56–75	1400–3700	28–47	700–2200	16–30	490–1300
6–12 yr	60–76	1200–2600	31–47	650–1500	18–35	370–1100
12–18 yr	56–84	1000–2200	31–52	530–1300	18–35	330–920

CD4 T-Cell Subpopulations						
CD4/CD45RA			**CD3/CD4/CD45RO**		**CD4/HLA-DR**	
Age	**Percent CD4 positive**	**Cells/mm³**	**Percent CD3/CD4 positive**	**Cells/mm³**	**Percent CD4 positive**	**Cells/mm³**
0–3 mo	64–95	1200–3700	2–22	60–900	2–6	40–180
3–6 mo	77–94	1300–3700	3–16	120–630	2–10	60–280
6–12 mo	64–93	1100–3700	5–18	160–800	2–11	50–260
1–2 yr	63–91	1000–2900	7–20	210–850	2–11	70–280
2–6 yr	53–86	430–1500	9–26	220–660	3–12	50–180
6–12 yr	46–77	320–1000	13–30	230–630	3–13	40–120
12–18 yr	33–66	230–770	18–38	240–700	4–11	30–100

CD8 T-Cell Subpopulations						
CD8/CD45RA			**CD3/CD4⁻/CD45RO**		**CD8/HLA-DR**	
Age	**Percent CD8 positive**	**Cells/mm³**	**Percent CD3/CD4 positive**	**Cells/mm³**	**Percent CD8 positive**	**Cells/mm³**
0–3 mo	80–99	450–1500	1–9	30–330	2–20	20–160
3–6 mo	85–98	550–1400	1–7	30–290	3–17	30–170
6–12 mo	75–97	480–1500	1–8	40–330	4–27	40–290
1–2 yr	71–98	490–1700	2–12	60–570	6–33	60–600
2–6 yr	69–97	380–1100	4–16	90–440	7–37	70–420
6–12 yr	63–92	310–900	4–21	70–390	6–29	40–270
12–18 yr	61–91	240–710	4–23	60–310	5–25	30–180

	B Cells and NK Cells			
	CD19		**CD3$^-$/CD16$^-$56$^+$**	
Age	**Percent positive**	**Cells/mm^3**	**Percent positive**	**Cells/mm^3**
0–3 mo	6–32	300–2000	4–18	170–1100
3–6 mo	11–41	430–3000	3–14	170–830
6–12 mo	14–37	610–2600	3–15	160–950
1–2 yr	16–35	720–2600	3–15	180–920
2–6 yr	14–33	390–1400	4–17	130–720
6–12 yr	13–27	270–860	4–17	100–480
12–18 yr	6–23	110–570	3–22	70–480

Data generated by Shearer WT, Rosenblatt HM, Gelman RS, Oyomopito R, Plaeger S, Stiehm ER, et al. Lymphocyte subsets in healthy children from birth through 18 years of age: the Pediatric AIDS Clinical Trials Group P1009 study. J Allergy Clin Immunol 2003;112(5):973–80.

REFERENCES

1. Piatosa B, Wolska-Kusnierz B, Pac M, Siewiera K, Gałkowska E, Bernatowska E. B cell subsets in healthy children: reference values for evaluation of B cell maturation process in peripheral blood. *Cytometry B Clin Cytom.* 2010;78(6):372–381.
2. Schatorje EJH, Gemen EFA, Driessen GJA, Leuvenink J, van Hout RW, de Vries E. Paediatric reference values for the peripheral T cell compartment. *Scan J Immunol.* 2012;75(4):436–444.
3. van Gent R, van Tilburg CM, Nibbelke EE, Otto SA, Gaiser JF, Janssens-Korpela PL, et al. Refined characterization and reference values of the pediatric T- and B-cell compartments. *Clin Immunol.* 2009; 133(1):95–107.

Index

Note: Page numbers followed by "f" indicate figures, "t" indicate tables and "b" indicate boxes

Printed and bound by CPI Group (UK) Ltd, Croydon, CR0 4YY

03/10/2024

01040373-0008